Spirituality, Health, and Healing

Caroline Young, MPH
ALLEGRA Learning Solutions, LLC
San Diego, California

Cyndie Koopsen, RN, MBA, HNC
ALLEGRA Learning Solutions, LLC
San Diego, California

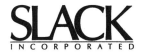

An innovative information, education, and management company
6900 Grove Road • Thorofare, NJ 08086

Printed in the United States of America.

Library of Congress Cataloging–in–Publication Data

Young, Caroline, MPH.
  Spirituality, health, and healing / Caroline Young, Cyndie Koopsen.
     p. ; cm.
  Includes bibliographical references and index.
  ISBN 1-55642-663-1 (alk. paper)
  1. Health--Religious aspects. 2. Spiritual healing. I. Koopsen, Cyndie. II. Title.
  BL65.M4Y68 2004
  201'.661--dc22

                                                                        2004013072

Published by: SLACK Incorporated
                  6900 Grove Road
                  Thorofare, NJ 08086 USA
                  Telephone: 856–848–1000
                  Fax: 856–853–5991
                  www.slackbooks.com

Contact SLACK Incorporated for more information about other books in this field or about the availability of our books from distributors outside the United States.
For permission to reprint material in another publication, contact SLACK Incorporated. Authorization to photocopy items for internal, personal, or academic use is granted by SLACK Incorporated provided that the appropriate fee is paid directly to Copyright Clearance Center. Prior to photocopying items, please contact the Copyright Clearance Center at 222 Rosewood Drive, Danvers, MA 01923 USA; phone: 978–750–8400; website: www.copyright.com; email: info@copyright.com

Last digit is print number: 10 9 8 7 6 5 4 3 2 1

DEDICATION

This book is dedicated to our families and friends,
whose love has supported, challenged, guided, and inspired us
to embrace our spiritual journey.

Contents

Dedication . . . . *v*

Acknowledgments . . . . *xi*

About the Authors . . . . *xiii*

Preface . . . . *xv*

Part I: The Spiritual Dimension

Chapter 1   Characteristics of Spirituality 3

                         Learning Objectives
                         Introduction

Learning Objectives
Introduction
The Spiritual Dimension
Theories of Spirituality
Defining Spirituality
Essential Elements of Spirituality
Spiritual Development
Spirituality and Healing
Summary
Key Concepts
Questions for Reflection
References

Chapter 2   Spirituality, the Health Care Professional,
                    and the Spiritual Care Provider 23

Learning Objectives
Introduction
Spiritual Health Care Providers
The Spirituality of Health Care Providers
Barriers to Providing Spiritual Care
Moral and Ethical Issues in Spiritual Care
Summary
Key Concepts
Questions for Reflection
References

Chapter 3   Spiritual Rituals 43

Learning Objectives
Introduction
Creating Rituals
Prayer
Meditation, Visualization, and Guided Imagery
Gratitude
Spending Time in Nature
Art
Storytelling
Rituals as a Healing Force
Summary
Key Concepts

Questions for Reflection
References

Chapter 4   Spirituality, Religion, and Health 59
              Learning Objectives
              Introduction
              Religion and Religiosity
              The Connection Between Spirituality, Religion, and Health
              The Benefits of Religion on Specific Health Conditions
              Religious Beliefs, Religious Practices, and Health
              Integrating Religious Practices and Beliefs Into Health Care
              Summary
              Key Concepts
              Questions for Reflection
              References

Chapter 5   Spirituality, Culture, and Health 75
              Learning Objectives
              Introduction
              Culture Defined
              How Are Spirituality, Culture, and Health Related?
              Compassion and Culturally Competent Care
              Looking Within: A Spiritual and Cultural Self-Assessment
              Health Belief Systems
              Health Care Systems
              Cultural Groups in the United States
              Language and Culturally Competent Care
              Summary
              Key Concepts
              Questions for Reflection
              References

Part II: Providing Spiritual Care

Chapter 6   Spiritual Assessment and Spiritual Care. 103
              Learning Objectives
              Introduction
              Spiritual Care
              Assessing Spiritual Status
              Preparing for the Spiritual Assessment: Strategies for Success
              Conducting the Spiritual Assessment
              Models for Spiritual Assessment
              Spiritual Diagnoses: Alterations in Spiritual Integrity
              Planning Spiritual Care
              Implementing Spiritual Care
              Evaluating Spiritual Care
              Summary
              Key Concepts
              Questions for Reflection
              References

Chapter 7   Therapeutic Interventions for Healing 125
                 Learning Objectives
                 Introduction
                 Music Therapy
                 Art Therapy
                 Dance and Movement Therapy
                 Humor Therapy
                 Animal-Assisted Therapy
                 Summary
                 Key Concepts
                 Questions for Reflection
                 References

Chapter 8   Spiritually Healing Environments. 147
                 Learning Objectives
                 Introduction
                 What Is a Spiritually Healing Environment?
                 A Shift in Focus
                 The Power of Design
                 Creating a Spiritually Healing Environment
                 The Health Care Provider as a Healing Environment
                 Summary
                 Key Concepts
                 Questions for Reflection
                 References

Part III: The Spiritual Dimension in End-of-Life Care

Chapter 9   Spiritual Care of the Dying 169
                 Learning Objectives
                 Introduction
                 Spiritual, Psychological, and Social Dimensions at the End of
                     Life
                 Cultural Considerations at the End of Life
                 Spiritual Caregiving Strategies
                 Hospice and Palliative Care
                 Advantages and Disadvantages of Dying at Home
                 Summary
                 Key Concepts
                 Questions for Reflection
                 References

Chapter 10   Spirituality and the Grieving Process 187
                 Learning Objectives
                 Introduction
                 The Grieving Process
                 Types of Grief Responses
                 Normal Grief Responses
                 Cultural Differences in Response to Grief
                 Coping With Grief

Grief Counseling and Elements of Healing
Summary
Key Concepts
Questions for Reflection
References

Part IV: Spirituality and Special Populations

Chapter 11   Spirituality, Religion, and Children 203
                  Learning Objectives
                  Introduction
                  The Development of Spirituality and Religion in Children
                  Phases of Psychosocial and Spiritual Development
                  Spiritual Assessments of Children
                  Spiritual Distress in Children
                  Providing Spiritual Care to Children
                  Spiritual Care of the Child With a Chronic Illness
                  Spiritual Care of the Dying Child
                  Summary
                  Key Concepts
                  Questions for Reflection
                  References

Chapter 12   Spiritual Dimensions of Aging 221
                  Learning Objectives
                  Introduction
                  The Unique Spiritual Challenges of Aging
                  A Changing Paradigm
                  Aging and the Human Spirit
                  Spiritual Development in the Aging Individual
                  Loss, Hope, Spirituality, and Aging
                  Love, Sexuality, Spirituality, and Aging
                  Religion, Spirituality, Aging, and Health
                  Coping Strategies for Difficult Times
                  Spiritual Interventions for the Aging Adult
                  Spiritual Elders
                  Summary
                  Key Concepts
                  Questions for Reflection
                  References

Index 241

ACKNOWLEDGMENTS

Our lives have been blessed with many wonderful relationships that have contributed immeasurably to the creation of this book. Our inspiration has come from many sources, including friends, family, and professional relationships. Some of those individuals are no longer with us in earthly forms, but they continue to guide and inspire us from their own special place. We are aware that there are many other individuals who helped us with this book but whose names are too numerous to mention. Their support, challenge, love, and unique gifts allowed this book to come into being, and we gratefully acknowledge their contribution.

We are grateful to all of those at SLACK Incorporated who believed in our project and provided unwavering support. Thank you Amy McShane and John Bond. You are a pleasure to work with.

We are incredibly blessed to know Gail Fink, a wonderful colleague and a calming presence during the creation of this book. Gail provided invaluable editorial expertise and words of wisdom during the development of this project. She is an amazing woman and we are grateful to know her and call her "friend." Thank you Gail. We could not have done it without you.

We want to express our immense gratitude and love for our families and for the sacrifices they have made as we undertook this adventure. They provided encouragement, guidance, inspiration, and examples of how amazing the gift of love can be along our spiritual journeys.

Caroline: To my husband Ron—although you are watching me from beyond, you nurtured my spirit and inspired me to realize my dreams. I will always keep close to my heart your extraordinary courage in living life. You were always the wind beneath my wings. To my children, Gina and Michael—your ongoing encouragement, faith in me, and unyielding love allowed me to reach incredible heights on my spiritual journey.

Cyndie: To Michael—thank you for always believing in me. You are my special gift in this life. Your love and support mean so very much and I am incredibly grateful for all you give to me. To my parents—words cannot begin to express how blessed I feel to be your daughter. You are two of the most amazing individuals in this world. Thank you for always "being there" and for encouraging and inspiring me to "reach for the stars" and be true to who I am.

Without you, our book would not have come into being.

Lastly, we'd like to acknowledge each other. We are incredibly lucky to be business partners and best friends. To be able to write, create, and experience all of this with each other has been a fabulous experience. We look forward to what comes next!

ABOUT THE AUTHORS

Our journey began almost 15 years ago when we first started working together in the community health and wellness department of a large metropolitan hospital. We instantly "connected" with each other and began a marvelous and deeply satisfying business partnership. We found we shared a mutual interest in other cultures and the spiritual aspects of care that were not well addressed in the health care environment in which we practiced.

In 1994, we founded ALLEGRA Learning Solutions, LLC, to provide print and online professional education courses for nurses and other health care professionals. Our journey took us down many interesting paths. We integrated our knowledge in the business we created through unique cultural and spiritual experiences with others. We have traveled extensively throughout the world and found our lives enriched by the many cultures and spiritual traditions we were privileged to share and the wonderful people we met along the way. Through sharing spiritual experiences with others, attending workshops and courses, and through personal spiritual study, we have broadened our understanding of the spiritual nature in all of us.

Our lives continue to teach us that our spiritual dimensions are an integral part of our entire being and a vital part of our health and healing. As we wrote this book, we discovered new dimensions to our beliefs as well as our relationship with ourselves, others, and our Higher Power.

Caroline Young, MPH, holds a Bachelor's degree in Psychology and a Master of Public Health degree with an emphasis in health promotion. Her extensive public health background includes expertise in research, design, development, marketing, implementation, and evaluation of community health programs. She also has expertise in developing education and health promotion programs for culturally diverse populations, senior populations, and faith communities.

Cyndie Koopsen, RN, MBA, HNC, is a registered nurse with a certification in public health and holistic nursing and a Master of Business Administration degree. Her professional nursing career has involved caring for clients in many settings and from many walks of life. In addition, she has managed large-scale clinical preventive programs and designed, developed, and presented educational programs for multicultural audiences covering the entire spectrum of health promotion and disease prevention.

Both Caroline and Cyndie have served as adjunct faculty members with several colleges and have coauthored distance education texts in the areas of cultural diversity, alternative medicine, and gerontology. They have conducted workshops, led seminars, and given presentations on numerous health care topics. They have developed more than 150 online professional continuing education courses and more than 100 distance education courses for vocational, baccalaureate, and master's level degree programs. They have also designed and developed certificate programs in the areas of spirituality, complementary and alternative medicine, gerontology, and end-of-life issues.

PREFACE

We wrote *Spirituality, Health, and Healing* to provide students, health care providers, and spiritual care providers with a comprehensive, unique resource for delivering effective, compassionate spiritual care to their current and future clients. This book is the result of our extensive training, research, and experience in the fields of nursing, psychology, public health, and education as well as direct clinical, research, writing, and consulting experience in the areas of spirituality and health.

Individuals, groups of students, and seasoned professionals in disciplines such as nursing, medicine, social work, physical therapy, occupational therapy, psychology, and theology can use this book. It is an excellent resource for clinical and classroom instructors alike and is a valuable addition to any instructor's library.

The content of this book is organized into four parts:

I. **The Spiritual Dimension:** As a foundation for the remainder of the text, the first section explores the spiritual dimension of individuals. This section examines the characteristics of spirituality; spirituality and the care provider; spiritual rituals; the connection between religion, spirituality, and health; and spirituality, culture, and health.

II. **Providing Spiritual Care:** The second section discusses the specific tools available to the health care professional in providing compassionate, effective spiritual care. Specifically, this section discusses spiritual assessment, therapeutic interventions, healing environments, spiritual evaluation, health care professionals, and spiritual care providers.

III. **The Spiritual Dimensions in End-of-Life Care:** The third section touches on the spiritual dimensions of this particular type of care, focusing on the spiritual care of the dying, hospice and palliative care, and spirituality and the grieving process.

IV. **Spirituality and Special Populations:** Finally, the fourth section explores the spiritual considerations of special populations, such as children and the aging individual.

Each section is organized into chapters. Each chapter can be used independently of the others. The beginning of each chapter contains learning objectives, and the end of each chapter contains a summary, key concepts, questions for reflection, and references. Shaded boxes highlight case studies and additional topics of interest.

An instructor's manual is available at http://www.efacultylounge.com. The manual contains individual, group, and community projects for classroom use.

PART I

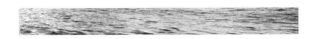

THE SPIRITUAL DIMENSION

Part I lays the foundation for *Spirituality, Health, and Healing* by exploring the spiritual dimension in individuals. This section examines:

- The characteristics of spirituality
- The relationship between spirituality, the health care professional, and the spiritual care provider
- Spiritual rituals
- The connection between religion, spirituality, and health
- The connection between spirituality, culture, and health

1

CHARACTERISTICS OF SPIRITUALITY

"We are not human beings on a spiritual journey,
but spiritual beings on a human journey."
—Pierre Teilhard de Chardin

LEARNING OBJECTIVES

Upon completing this chapter, you will be able to do the following:
1. Explain theories of spirituality.
2. Compare the definitions of spirituality.
3. Describe the essential elements of spirituality.
4. List and explain the stages of spiritual development.
5. Describe the connection between spirituality and healing.

INTRODUCTION

Over the last several decades, the topic of spirituality has come to the forefront of public and professional consciousness. With the dawn of a new century, spirituality has received increased coverage in the media and more discussion in the workplace, politics, and education (Messikomer & De Craemer, 2002). Spirituality has also become more apparent in health care, with increasing evidence that spiritual factors are important components of health and well-being (Dossey, 2001). The need for health care providers to effectively address the connection between spirituality and health is becoming widely recognized.

As the information age gives way to the intuition age, health care professionals will need to focus less on logical, linear, mechanical thinking and more on creative, lateral, emotional thinking (Reynolds, 2001). This shift in focus will require the provision of care to encompass a more holistic perspective—one that attends to all aspects of the mind, body, and spirit. As Burkhardt and Nagai-Jacobson (2002) so aptly write in their book, *Spirituality: Living Our Connectedness*, "Spirituality is at the heart of caring for the whole person" (p. 1).

Yet the lack of a clear definition or a concise conceptual framework, coupled with limited opportunities for spiritual training and professional development of health care providers, has resulted in the neglect of this aspect of client care. This book will attempt to help fill that gap, beginning with an exploration of the many theories and definitions of spirituality, the stages of spiritual development, and the connection between spirituality and healing.

Please Note

No discussion of spirituality would be complete without referring to the concept of a Higher Power or creator. This being is known throughout the world by many different names, including God, Goddess, Higher Power, Divine Spirit, Ultimate Being, the Absolute, Lord, Inner Light, Life Source, Allah, Tao, Spirit, the Way, and Universal Love. Because it would be too cumbersome to try to include all the different names on every use, we will most often use the term *God* throughout this book. We mean no disrespect to anyone and sincerely hope none is taken.

THE SPIRITUAL DIMENSION

Spirituality encompasses all aspects of being human and is a means of experiencing life. Spirituality has also been defined as an integral dimension of the health and well-being of every individual (Skokan & Bader, 2000). By caring for clients in a way that acknowledges the mind-body-spirit connection, health care providers acknowledge the whole person (Cobb & Robshaw, 1998; Goddard, 2000).

In the past, spiritual care was synonymous with religious care. Although spirituality may include traditional religious beliefs and practices (discussed in Chapter 4), spirituality is a much broader concept that also includes nonreligious beliefs and expressions (Thomason & Brody, 1999). Today's multicultural society, with its many secular and religious beliefs, requires spiritual care that respects the integrity of different faith communities as well as that of individuals outside the faith communities (Cobb & Robshaw, 1998).

Enblen (1992) examined the literature to determine the differences in definition regarding the concept of spirituality and religion. He found that the following six words appeared most frequently when describing religion: *system*, *beliefs*, *organized*, *person*, *worship*, and *practices*. In descriptions of spirituality, the following nine words appeared most frequently: *personal*, *life*, *principle*, *animator*, *being*, *God/god*, *quality*, *relationship*, and *transcendent*.

In the holistic perspective of health care, the mind, body, and spirit are interconnected and interact in a dynamic way in the "whole person," making it difficult and artificial to try to separate these three dimensions. However, health care providers find it useful to distinguish between them for purposes of assessment and treatment. One way to differentiate between them is the following (Mansen, 1993; Taylor, 2002):

- The **psychological dimension (mind)** involves self-consciousness and self-identity. It is that aspect of an individual that deals with issues related to human interactions (and associated emotions such as grief, loss, and guilt) on an intimate level.
- The **physical dimension (body)** is world-conscious. It is that aspect of an individual that allows him or her to taste, feel, see, hear, smell, and be experienced by others.
- The **spiritual dimension (spirit)** is described as a unifying force within an individual, integrating and transcending all other dimensions. This dimension is also described as God-consciousness, or related to a deity or supreme values. It is concerned with the meaning of life, individual perceptions of faith, and an individual's relationship with the Ultimate Being.

THEORIES OF SPIRITUALITY

Spirituality is reflected in everyday life as well as in disciplines ranging from philosophy and popular literature to psychotherapy, health psychology, medicine, nursing, sociology, and science (Chandler, 1999; Hatch, Burg, Naberhaus, & Hellmich, 1998; Mahoney & Graci, 1999; Tuck, Wallace, & Pullen, 2001).

While no one has been able to provide a universally accepted definition of spirituality, theorists and researchers agree that it is a multidimensional phenomenon, and descriptions of its characteristics are abundant in the literature. The theories presented here are samples of some of the theories in use today. They include concepts from theology, psychology, sociology, medicine, and nursing.

Theological, Psychological, and Sociological Theories

Theology describes spirituality as one's belief in God, which is expressed through religious beliefs and practices.

In psychology, spirituality is explained as an expression of one's internal motives and desires, concentrating on the self instead of God. Psychology examines one's spiritual search for meaning, purpose, and guidance.

Sociology examines the concept of spirituality by studying groups of people. According to sociology, people strongly influence other people, who are in turn influenced by the groups in which they live. Sociology describes spirituality as the spiritual practices and rituals of groups of people as well as the social morality within personal relationships (Meraviglia, 1999).

Medical Theories

Until recently, contemporary medicine has historically given little attention to the spiritual dimension despite its importance in the fundamental goal of healing. However, medicine now focuses increased attention on exploring the relationship between clients' spiritual needs and more traditional aspects of their medical care. Medical schools have begun offering courses in spirituality, religion, and health, with many schools receiving grants from the National Institute for Healthcare Research to develop curricula in spirituality and medicine (Hiatt, 1986; Koenig et al., 1999).

Trends that appear to be driving this new interest in spirituality include the many studies that have demonstrated a strong connection between spirituality and improved health, client demand for greater personal attention from their physicians, the growing importance of end-of-life care, and the increasing dissatisfaction among physicians with what they view as an increasingly depersonalized practice (Moran, 1999).

Nursing Theories

Nursing incorporates all the aforementioned perspectives (theology, psychology, sociology, and medicine) while also examining spirituality quantitatively from other perspectives, including spiritual health, spiritual well-being, spiritual perspective, self-transcendence, faith, quality of life, hope, religiousness, purpose in life, and spiritual coping (Meraviglia, 1999). Traditionally, nursing has always been concerned with the health care of the whole person, including the physical, psychological, social, cultural, environmental, and spiritual dimensions (Bergquist & King, 1994; Martsolf & Mickley, 1998).

Nursing theoretical models in which spirituality is a major concept include Betty Neuman's Neuman systems model, Margaret Newman's theory of health, Rosemary Parse's theory of human becoming, and Jean Watson's theory of human caring:

- Betty Neuman's **Neuman systems model** focuses on the wellness of the client in relationship to environmental stressors and reactions to stressors. In the Neuman systems model, the client/client system is described as the central core, surrounded by concentric rings. The central core includes innate energy resources or basic survival factors common to all people, and the rings are the mechanisms that protect the central core. The entire client system contains five variables: physiological, psychological, sociocultural, developmental, and spiritual. To address the wholeness concept of care, practitioners must consider all five variables. Several authors have expanded Neuman's model to include issues related to spiritual well-being, spiritual needs, spiritual care, and spiritual distress (Fawcett, 2001; Knight, 1990; Martsolf & Mickley, 1998).

- **Margaret Newman's theory of health** expanded Martha Rogers' idea of humans as energy fields to humans as unique patterns of consciousness. Newman's theory defines consciousness as the capacity of the system to interact with the environment, and Newman posited that the process of life involves movement toward higher levels of consciousness. The dimensions of person-environment interaction include exchanging, communicating, relating, valuing, choosing, moving, perceiving, feeling, and knowing. Newman described expanded consciousness as a general spiritual term (Martsolf & Mickley, 1998).

- **Rosemary Parse's theory of human becoming** was developed to move nursing's view of the person from the medical model to a human science perspective (Martsolf & Mickley, 1998; Parse, 1992). In their book, *Holistic Nursing: A Handbook for Practice*, Dossey, Keegan, and Guzzetta (2000) describe Parse's theory in the following way: "Person is a unified, whole being. Health is a process of becoming; it is a personal commitment, an unfolding, a process related to lived experiences. Environment is the universe. The human-universe is inseparable and evolving together" (p. 179).

- **Jean Watson's theory of human caring** is based on a spiritual-existential and phenomenological orientation that draws on Eastern philosophies. It focuses on nurse-client interactions and posits that humans are energy fields with patterns of consciousness. This theory acknowledges the spiritual dimension of people. In Watson's theory, caring is considered the essence of nursing practice and requires the nurse to be personally, morally, and spiritually engaged. The one caring and the one being cared for are considered coparticipants in self-healing; they each have the power to heal themselves (Falk-Rafael, 2000; Martsolf & Mickley, 1998; Saewyc, 2000; Watson, 1988).

For theoretical unity to be achieved, there is a need for consistency and universality in both the terminology and language used to describe the spiritual dimension (McSherry & Draper, 1998). The challenge for health care providers and spiritual care providers is to agree on such a universal theory. A universal, inclusive definition of the spiritual dimension that reflects the unique nature of all individuals will provide a basis for research and enable spirituality to be studied more carefully.

DEFINING SPIRITUALITY

Defying development of a standard definition, spirituality remains a highly subjective, personal, and individualistic concept (Coyle, 2002). To many, spirituality represents a necessary essence of life that energizes both thoughts and actions (Taylor, 2002). To others, spirituality is a belief in a power operating in the universe greater than one's self. Still others define it as a sense of interconnectedness with all living creatures and an awareness of the purpose and meaning of life (Walton, 1999).

Universal Definitions

Although the definitions vary on some points, they seem to agree that all people are spiritual beings. Each person has a spiritual dimension that motivates, energizes, and influences every aspect of his or her life.

Spirituality can be considered a basic human quality that transcends gender, race, color, and national origin. At the same time, spirituality has many intangible aspects and is an intensely personal issue. It means different things to different people, and these differences are often difficult to describe. Many individuals cannot describe "a spiritual experience," yet they are convinced that they have experienced something spiritual (Taylor, 2002).

The term *spirituality* is derived from the Latin *spiritus*, meaning breath. It is also related to the Greek *pneuma*, or breath, which refers to the vital spirit or soul. According to Dossey et al. (2000), spirituality is the essence of who and how people are in the world and, like breathing, is essential to human existence. Miller (1995), in an article titled "Culture, Spirituality, and Women's Health," further elaborates, "If one believes that spirituality permeates all human experiences rather than being additional to them, one must accept it as integral to health or a sense of wholeness or well-being" (p. 258).

In *Spiritual Care*, Taylor (2002) notes that dictionaries define spirituality through a variety of terms, including the following:
- Sacred
- Moral

- Holy or divine
- Of pure essence
- Intellectual and higher endowments of the mind
- Ecclesiastical (relating to religious organizations)
- Incorporeal (without a physical dimension)
- Spirits or supernatural entities
- Highly refined in thought and feeling

A consensus panel of experts at the National Institute of Healthcare Research also attempted to define spirituality. Following an extensive review of research on spirituality and religion, the panel defined spirituality as "the feelings, thoughts, experiences, and behaviors that arise from a search for the sacred" (Boudreaux, O'Hea, & Chasuk, 2002, p. 439).

Additional sources provide their own definitions for spirituality:

- **Spirituality involves the nonphysical, immaterial aspects** of an individual's being with energies, essences, and the parts of people that will exist after their bodies disintegrate. The whole picture of health involves physical, mental, and spiritual components. Whether or not a person is religious, he or she can lead a spiritual life and explore the influence of spirituality on health (Weil, 1997).
- **Spirituality is the animation force, life principle, or essence of being** that permeates life and is expressed and experienced in multifaceted connections with the self, others, nature, and God or life force. Shaped by cultural experiences, spirituality is a universal human experience (Miller, 1995).
- **Spirituality is rooted in an awareness** that is part of the biological makeup of the human species. Spirituality is present in all individuals and it may manifest as inner peace and strength derived from a perceived relationship with a transcendent God, an ultimate reality, or whatever an individual values as supreme (Narayanasamy, 1999).

Spiritual Issues

In *Core Curriculum for Holistic Nursing*, Dossey (1997) defines spiritual issues as "core life issues" that cannot be quantified and often have no clear answers. Dossey's list of spiritual issues includes the following:

- **Mystery:** That which cannot be understood or explained.
- **Suffering:** Why mind, body, and spiritual pain are present and what they mean.
- **Forgiveness:** The choice to release one's self or another from judgment because of a perceived wound.
- **Grace:** An understanding of the gifts of life that are often attributed to providence.
- **Hope:** Desire accompanied by expectation of fulfillment.
- **Love:** An acknowledged mystery that is experienced and expressed in caring acts, both given and received.

Health Care Definitions

Health care providers need to be concerned about a client's spirituality because it provides insight into the client's experience, provides a context for making health care decisions, and allows health care professionals to help clients in a way that limits suffering. Within the health care profession, the following additional concepts help define spirituality (Burkhardt, 1989; Dyson, Cobb, & Forman, 1997; Taylor, 2002):

- **Inspiriting:** The ever-evolving, interconnected, harmonious "mystery" that arises from an individual's inner strength. How a person responds to life events determines his or her "spirit titer" and will result in that individual either being uplifted (inspirited) or disheartened (dispirited).
- **Spiritual quality of life:** A phrase suggesting that an individual's spiritual dimension is crucial to a quality life; strong beliefs, hope, religiosity, and inner strength contribute to a meaningful life
- **Spiritual well-being:** A term often found in nursing literature, spiritual well-being identifies harmonious interconnectedness with a deity, the self, the community, and the environment. It also relates to life-affirming relationships, creative energy, the wholeness of an individual's spirit and unifying dimension of health, faith in a higher power, enhancement of the individual's inner resources, and inner strength.
- **Spiritual disequilibrium:** A state of inner chaos that occurs when an individual's most cherished beliefs are challenged. This frequently occurs during the time when a life-threatening illness is diagnosed.
- **Spiritual need, spiritual problem, spiritual concern:** A factor determined by a specific individual to be necessary to establish or maintain the individual's relationship with his or her Higher Power. Spiritual needs have been described as the deepest requirement of the self.
- **Spiritual distress:** A disruption of life principles that pervades every aspect of a person's being and transcends the biological and psychosocial aspects of that person's nature.
- **Spiritual pain, spiritual alienation, spiritual anxiety, anger, guilt, loss, and despair:** Specific nursing diagnoses that describe an individual who has a pervasive loneliness of spirit, often stemming from an intense feeling of alienation from his or her God or Higher Power and manifested by a deep sense of hurt.

ESSENTIAL ELEMENTS OF SPIRITUALITY

To properly identify their clients' spiritual needs and provide spiritual care, health care providers must understand the elements of spirituality and how they are expressed by different individuals.

A review of the literature explores the meaning of spirituality and reveals that:

> ...the self, others, and 'God' provide the key elements within a definition of spirituality and that other emerging themes, namely meaning and purpose, hope, relatedness/connectedness, beliefs/belief systems, and expressions of spirituality, can be articulated in the context of those three key elements. (Dyson et al., 1997, p. 1183)

The key elements of spirituality are discussed below.

Self, Others, and God

The centrality of the relationships between self, others, and a Higher Power or God is a major focus of spirituality and a prominent emerging theme in the spiritual literature.

- **Self:** The individual's inner self and inner resources are fundamental in the exploration of spirituality.
- **Others:** The individual's relationships with others are equally important. The need for affiliation and interdependence has long been recognized as part of the human experience.
- **God:** The concept of God and a person's relationship with God have traditionally been understood within a religious framework. Today, however, a broader and less restrictive framework is emerging. God is experienced as a unifying force, life principle, or essence of being. The nature of God may take many forms and have different meanings for different individuals. Individuals experience God in many ways, such as in relationships, nature, music, art, and pets. For example, nurturing children or caring for plants and animals can provide a sense of self-satisfaction and joy (Walton, 1999). Effective health care providers and spiritual care providers integrate these expressions of spirituality in their care of clients.

Spiritual relationships with self, others, and a Higher Power can be a tremendous source of comfort, providing healing energy and strength to an individual. This energy can be reciprocal, insightful, and meaningful for both health care providers and clients (Dyson et al., 1997; Walton, 1996).

Meaning and Purpose

Another essential element of spirituality is finding meaning and purpose in life (Burkhardt & Nagai-Jacobson, 2002). The quest to find meaning in life emerges as a dominant theme in spirituality, with the relationship to self, others, and God contributing to its discovery (Dyson et al., 1997). In *The Meaning of Everyday Occupation*, Hasselkus (2002) states:

So, where do meanings come from? They are personally and socially derived. For some, meanings in life may be heavily weighted by personal and unique values and histories; for others, meanings may stem largely from the community and culture in which we live. From a life span perspective, the sources of meaning in our lives may be thought of as a continuum or as a developmental trajectory that unfolds throughout life. (p. 3)

Burkhardt (1989) describes this search for meaning as an "unfolding mystery." The need for purpose and meaning in life is a universal trait and may be essential to life itself. If an individual is unable to find meaning and purpose, all aspects of his or her life may be affected and a sense of emptiness and unworthiness can result. Spiritual distress may then be experienced, which can contribute to emotional distress and can ultimately lead to physical problems (Burkhardt & Nagai-Jacobson, 2002).

Spiritual individuals experience more meaning or purpose in life than do their nonspiritual counterparts. Some individuals are able to derive meaning from an adverse experience in such a way that it promotes a sense of well-being or healing (Mahoney & Graci, 1999). Meaning in life is an outcome of spirituality that can be effectively measured and can be found creatively through poetry or painting, adherence to a political ideology, or in relationships with other people (Goldberg, 1998; Meraviglia, 1999).

Hope

Hope, spiritual need common to everyone, can be described as a sense of energy exchanged between individuals and their environment. It is perceived as emanating from mutual affiliation and concern for others as well as the self, and it encompasses a sense of relatedness to possibilities and powers beyond the self and the present (Hinds, 1988; Owen, 1989).

Spiritual individuals tend to be more hopeful than their nonspiritual peers (Mahoney & Graci, 1999). It is often said that where there is life, there is hope, but Kleindienst (1998) also believes that there is just as much truth to the opposite sentiment: Where there is hope, there is life.

Relatedness/Connectedness

The term *connection* implies a joining together of two or more elements, with a relationship formed between them (Goldberg, 1998). Burkhardt (1989) describes this sense of relatedness and connectedness in terms of harmony—harmony with the self and others, and a sense of relatedness to God.

Dyer (2001) acknowledges in his book, *There's a Spiritual Solution to Every Problem*, the innate interconnectedness of people with each other: "At the level of spiritual consciousness we know we are connected to everyone" (p. 14). Dossey (1997) offers the following examples of this interconnectedness:

- Loving, painful, supportive, and difficult relationships with family, friends, and others.
- Caring for others and being cared for by others.
- Recognizing relationships as a source of growth and change.

Spirituality is intertwined with every aspect of life and provides purpose, meaning, strength, and guidance in shaping the journey of life. As Dyer (2001) writes, "Spirituality is from within, the result of recognition, realization, and reverence" (p. 10). Or, as Dossey (1997) says, "spirituality can be experienced in the mundane as well as in the profound."

Spirituality also involves relationships with someone or something beyond the self. That someone or something can sustain and comfort us, guide our decision making, forgive our imperfections, and celebrate our journey through life (Spaniol, 2002).

Spirituality is also expressed and experienced through interconnectedness with nature, the earth, the environment, and the cosmos. All life exists in an interconnected web; what happens to the earth affects everyone, and everyone's behavior affects the earth. Therefore, it is essential to be aware of and to appreciate the interconnected web of all life. Spirituality contributes to this awareness and appreciation (Dossey, 1997; Spaniol, 2002).

Spaniol (2002) writes, "Connectedness is what is authentic for us—what is natural and spontaneous. To be connected is to be an integrated, mutual, contributing partner in the world we live in." The consequences of disconnectedness (from self, others, and a larger meaning or God) can include self-alienation, loneliness, and a lack of meaning or purpose (Bellingham, Cohen, Jones, & Spaniol, 1989).

Beliefs and Belief Systems

Still another essential element of spirituality is the concept of beliefs and belief systems. Dossey et al. (2000) describe *beliefs* as "a subclass of attitudes. The cognitive factors involved in beliefs have less to do with facts and more with feelings; they represent a personal confidence or faith in the validity of some person, object, or idea" (p. 56). Faith can be an important part of an individual's beliefs and decisions in life. Faith may be described as a belief in God, an almighty being, or a Higher Power that gives meaning and purpose in life. Developing faith is an active and ongoing process and is unique to each individual, embedded with the past, present, and hopes of the future (Carson, 1989).

For some, spiritual beliefs are exclusively related to religion, while they may not be related at all for others. Widespread evidence shows that the interest in spirituality is not confined to individuals who attend church or who are identified as religious people (Shea, 2000). Dyson et al. (1997) state that if God is defined as the construct that represents the principal value in a person's life and which patterns and shapes the person's beliefs, values, and choices, then both religious and nonreligious belief systems should be considered in the exploration of spirituality.

If the health care profession is to establish a definition and provide a conceptual framework of spirituality that encompasses the needs of all its clients, this narrow and restrictive view of relating the concept to religion must be expanded. Religion is more about systems of practices and beliefs within which social groups engage. This is not to say that religion has no part to play in spirituality for some people. Spirituality is simply a broader concept (Dyson et al., 1997).

The essential elements of spirituality—such as transcendence, meaning and purpose, connectedness, hope, and faith—work to produce health benefits in terms of prevention, recovery from illness, and coping with illness. Health care practitioners who actively explore the content of the belief systems of their clients in a respectful manner can better appreciate the benefits clients might experience from their belief and value systems (Coyle, 2002). Health care providers should also be aware of, and know the importance of, their own belief systems as well as those of others (Dossey et al., 2000).

Expressions of Spirituality

Spirituality can be expressed through rituals such as prayer, meditation, guided imagery, visualization, practicing gratitude, spending time in nature, viewing and engaging in art, and storytelling (discussed in Chapter 3). Spirituality can also be expressed through questioning. As Streeter (1996) writes:

> Humans' most basic spiritual activity is questioning. We question our experience itself; we question our understanding of the experience. We question whether our understanding is correct, and finally, we question what we need to do about what we know to be true. (p. 17)

For health care providers to adequately assess a client's spirituality and provide appropriate spiritual care, they must be sensitive to the various ways in which spirituality may be expressed and experienced. They must also recognize and properly interpret common manifestations of spirituality. These manifestations are usually most obvious when someone has a spiritual need, including the need to (Goldberg, 1998; Taylor, 2002):

- Have meaning and purpose
- Have hope
- Give and receive love
- Express feelings
- Have connections
- Relate to or worship a Supreme Being
- Forgive or be forgiven

SPIRITUAL DEVELOPMENT

According to Hiatt (1986), spiritual development is individualistic and involves a series of steps or cycles that occur in no particular order or timeframe throughout the life of an individual. Much like physical or psychological development, spiritual development may follow an uneven, stepwise course.

- The first half of life is comprised of ego development.
- In midlife, the individual begins to sense that the ego is superficial and begins to shift his or her identity to the true "self" (i.e., the part of the person that is not contingent on specific life history and choices). This self is the psychological representation of spirit, and it is during this period that people are most likely to become consciously spiritual.

Awareness of spirituality is often triggered by life experiences, such as having a child, experiencing an illness, facing the prospect of one's own death or the death of another, or confronting a crisis in a personal relationship. Additional experiences that may contribute to or serve to initiate spiritual awareness can include praying, engaging in physical exercise, listening to music, gazing at art, and being alone (Meraviglia, 1999).

Fowler's Stages of Faith Development

Spiritual development is just as possible as physical, intellectual, emotional, or moral development. After interviewing more than 400 people ranging from 3 to 84 years of age, Fowler (1987) proposed seven stages of faith development. Fowler's linear theory of faith development attempts to identify the dynamic process by which human beings find meaning in life and a purpose for their existence. Although it is typically associated with religious faith, Fowler recognized faith as a universal phenomenon.

The following is a summary of Fowler's stages of faith development (Carson, 1989; Fowler, 1987; Taylor, 2002):

- **Stage 0: Undifferentiated faith** (infancy to 3 years of age)—a period during which infants and toddlers acquire the fundamental qualities of faith, trust, mutuality, and love.
- **Stage 1: Intuitive-projective faith** (3 to 7 years of age)—a period during which children are influenced by stories, examples, moods, and actions of visible faith, usually displayed in the home.
- **Stage 2: Mythic-literal faith** (usually up to 12 years of age but can extend into adulthood)—a period during which children try to sort out fantasy and fact. They often demand "proof" of reality and interpret stories literally. They begin to realize that they belong to a community beyond the home.

- **Stage 3: Synthetic-conventional faith** (usually adolescence but can extend into adulthood)—a period during which the individual reflects on the incongruities of the stories. Individuals conform to the beliefs of those around them because they have not yet learned to view others objectively.
- **Stage 4: Individuative-reflective faith** (usually young adults but can extend into later adulthood)—a period during which a self-identity and worldview are differentiated from others' identities and views. Independent lifestyles, beliefs, and attitudes form during this stage.
- **Stage 5: Conjunctive faith** (adults past midlife)—a period in which adults find a new appreciation for their past, value their inner voices, and become aware of deep-seated myths and prejudices due to their social background. Individuals who reach this stage do not try to "convert" someone of another faith. Instead, they embrace persons of other faith traditions and try to glean new understandings from them. They are involved in listening to their deeper self instead of praying for specific things or events.
- **Stage 6: Universalizing faith** (midlife or beyond)—a stage that is infrequently reached since individuals at this stage are committed visionaries. Examples include Mahatma Gandhi and Mother Teresa. With passion and yet some detachment, individuals who reach this stage continue to spend themselves in love, devoted to overcoming division, oppression, and violence. They become actualizers of the spirit of an inclusive human community.

It must be noted that Fowler's theory of faith development is grounded in the experience of Western culture. Although the influence of Western culture is widespread, it is not universal. For that reason, Fowler's stage theory of faith development may not apply to other religious and spiritual worldviews. For example, it cannot explain the spiritual growth of a primitive shaman, an Islamic fundamentalist, or cognitively impaired individuals (because of its dependence on verbal ability). It does not explain the Eastern view of spiritual development in which the integration of mind and body with the universal divine spirit unfolds in a cyclic manner and is achieved through a series of incarnations (Macrae, 2001).

Spiritual Growth

According to Carson (1989) and McSherry and Draper (1998), spiritual growth involves a two-directional process. The horizontal process increases an individual's awareness of the transcendent values inherent in all relationships and activities of life. It reflects a person's beliefs, values, lifestyle, and the human environmental elements and interactions of existence. The vertical process involves promoting a closer relationship with a Higher Being as conceived by the individual.

The horizontal process may develop without the vertical process developing. For example, spiritual growth may progress in terms of relationships, art, or music but may never evolve into a relationship with a Higher Being. Conversely, individuals may develop a relationship with a Higher Being and may never develop other forms of spiritual expression.

SPIRITUALITY AND HEALING

Burkhardt and Nagai-Jacobson (2002) write, "Healing and spirituality are intimately connected. Grounded in the understanding that spirituality is the essence of who we are as human beings, we believe that healing is essentially a spiritual process that attends to the wholeness of a person" (p. 25).

A little over a decade ago, hardly any information existed on the relationship between spirituality and health. Now there is a tremendous amount of research on the meaning of spirituality as well as the appropriate methods for assessment and the implications of that assessment on client care (Draper & McSherry, 2002).

Since 1991, the National Institute for Healthcare Research has reviewed studies that examine the influence of spirituality on health (Larson, Swyers, & McCullough, 1998). These studies looked at the effects of spirituality on the likelihood of dying from conditions such as respiratory disease, cancer, and heart disease. Most studies compared individuals who participated in religious activities to those who did not, and the studies found that religious or spiritual people lived longer. This effect was seen in both men and women from different age groups, religions, ethnic groups, and countries. Many individuals believe their spirituality helps promote healing, especially in cases in which medications and other treatments cannot provide a cure for their conditions.

The success of 12-step programs such as Alcoholics Anonymous also provides direct evidence of the potential power of spirituality on medical conditions. Indeed, hospice programs and Alcoholics Anonymous are some of the strongest supporters of providing clients with spiritual care (Hatch et al., 1998). With mounting evidence of the link between spirituality and healing, this is an area that needs and deserves closer examination.

What Is Healing?

Spirituality and healing are intimately connected. *Healing* is a spiritual process that attends to the wholeness of an individual. It occurs over time, continuing through the individual's life journey and becoming a way of living that flows from, reflects, and nourishes his or her spirit (Burkhardt & Nagai-Jacobson, 2002).

It is important to understand the difference between "healing" and "curing." *Curing* is physical, alleviating the signs and symptoms of disease at the anatomical level. *Healing*, in contrast, is spiritual, intangible, and experiential, involving an integration of body, mind, and spirit. Curing is concerned with wholeness of body, while healing is concerned with wholeness of being (Skokan & Bader, 2000). Healing and curing can occur together or separately. An individual can be healed without being cured or cured without being healed.

Cultures from around the world offer various models for understanding the relationship between spirituality, healing, and illness. For more than 100,000 years and still today in many cultures, the knowledge of healing has been held by shamans or medicine people who attend to the well-being of their communities. Long before Western science-based practices existed, cultural healers helped people. Today, about 70% to 90% of the people worldwide turn to practitioners of nonallopathic traditions of practice. These healers blend the functions of healing with spiritual leadership (Miller, 1999). For example, the Navajos believe the natural state of all things in creation, including the human person, is one of harmony. Having a disease or an illness indicates disharmony, and Navajo healing rituals focus on restoring harmony within the person and between the person, the spirit world, the community, and the environment. A Navajo healing ceremony includes the family and community, and its goal is to restore a sense of connectedness within the person's life, relationships, and environment (Burkhardt & Nagai-Jacobson, 2002).

The complex connections between religious and spiritual beliefs and practices and an individual's physical and psychological health are only just beginning to be explored. Researchers have discovered a positive relationship between religion and physical and mental health and have demonstrated that spiritual beliefs and practices are beneficial to health and can help reduce the risk of developing a number of serious illnesses (Ebersole & Hess, 1997; Larson et al., 1998).

As a result of these discoveries, health care professionals are beginning to examine their own spirituality as well as that of their clients, learn about the world's major religious teachings, learn how to take a spiritual history, and better communicate with clients about their spiritual concerns.

Spiritual Well-Being

Spiritual well-being is the ability to find meaning, value, and purpose in life and thus to feel content, fulfilled, and happy (Burkhardt & Nagai-Jacobson, 2002). It also relates to life-affirming relationships, creative energy, the wholeness of an individual's spirit and unifying dimension of health, faith in a Higher Power, enhancement of the individual's inner resources, and inner strength.

Spiritual well-being is a "present state of peace and harmony... linked to past experiences and future hopes and goals" (Hungelmann, Kenkel-Rossi, Klassen, & Stollenwerk, 1985, p. 151). According to Pilch (1988), wellness involves holistic spirituality. An individual can be near death or be mentally or physically disabled and still possess "wellness spirituality." Spiritual wellness is a way of life that views life and living as purposeful and pleasurable. It has roots in spiritual values and/or specific religious beliefs and it involves life-sustaining and life-enriching options that are selected freely at every opportunity.

Humanistic psychologist Abraham Maslow is well known for developing his hierarchy of needs. He theorized that people progress from basic needs (e.g., safety, food, and shelter) to higher needs of social interaction and self-worth. Spiritual well-being parallels Maslow's highest stage, self-actualization, in which the individual possesses the ability to "extend the self beyond boundaries of the immediate context and achieve new perspectives and experiences" (Leetun, 1996, p. 60).

Spiritual well-being has also been associated with satisfaction with life; productivity; happiness; an increased energy level; and physical, emotional, and mental well-being (Isaia, Parker, & Murrow, 1999). High-level wellness results from an integration of the mind, body, and spirit in conjunction with maximum functioning within an existing environment (Leetun, 1996).

Spiritual well-being is an indication of an individual's quality of life in the spiritual dimension. According to Fehring, Miller, and Shaw (1997), spiritual well-being has two components: a vertical dimension that involves a relationship with a Higher Being or God and a horizontal dimension that involves a sense of purpose and meaning in life. Spiritual well-being is not synonymous with belief or practice in the particular aspects of a religion. Instead, it is an affirmation of life in a relationship with God, self, community, and environment. It nurtures wholeness (Blazer, 1991).

Blazer (1991) defined six dimensions of spiritual well-being in his article "Spirituality and Aging Well":

1. **Self-determined wisdom:** A knowledge of the larger system in which one lives and the ability to understand and accept the limits of that environment so the balance of the system is maintained.
2. **Self-transcendence:** The ability to cross the boundary beyond the self.
3. **Meaning:** The ability to evaluate the meaning of one's life in light of the losses and the totality of one's life experiences.
4. **Accepting the totality of life:** An understanding that there is no changing of one's life course in retrospect and that there is only one life to live.
5. **Revival of spirituality:** A resurgence of the spirituality that may have been abandoned during the younger years.
6. **Exit and existence:** The understanding that death and dying are inevitable; the shift to a positive outlook on aging (rather than a negative one).

Spiritual Health

Spiritual well-being not only indicates an individual's quality of life in the spiritual dimension, but it is also an indication of spiritual health. According to Chapman (1987):

> Spiritual health may be considered as the ability to develop our spiritual nature to its fullest potential. This would include our ability to discover and articulate our own basic purpose in life, learn how to experience love, joy, peace and fulfillment and how to help others and ourselves achieve their full potential. (p. 32)

Being spiritually healthy means being connected to a spouse, partner, family, friends, and community. It means having the ability to live in the wholeness of life (Bellingham et al., 1989). Spiritual health leads to a heightened awareness of the Divine Spirit referred to by all religions. It isn't important whether the being is called God, Allah, Buddha, Spirit, Higher Power, or any other name; what matters is the awareness of the role the Divine Spirit plays in the individual's life (Reynolds, 2001).

Self-care approaches that include prayer, meditation, gratitude, spending time in nature, rest and leisure, and art can deepen one's spiritual awareness and enhance one's spiritual health (Reynolds, 2001). Observing spiritual and religious traditions by working with spiritual counselors and support groups is also a method of enhancing spiritual health.

Healing and Spiritual Presence

Spiritual health is often overlooked in the process of healing, but one of the most important ways to integrate spiritual care into health care is simply by being present with the client. According to Burkhardt and Nagai-Jacobson (2002), "Spiritual care begins with presence" (p. 86). They add, "When we encounter another at the level of spirit, we open to the sacredness of the present moment" (p. 87). Presence can be named loving presence, therapeutic presence, caring presence, transpersonal presence, transcendent presence, and intentional presence. It can include listening, feeling close, sensing, speaking, sitting with, touching, empathizing, supporting, attending, and attentively giving physical care (Burkhardt & Nagai-Jacobson, 2002; Zerwekh, 1997).

Burkhardt and Nagai-Jacobson (2002) continue, "Because the essential nature of these various understandings of presence flows from our spiritual core, we consider the essence of healing presence to be spiritual presence" (p. 86). Resulting in personal and professional growth of both the health care provider and the client, being present requires deliberate focused attention, receptivity of the individual, and awareness of a shared humanity (Zerwekh, 1997).

SUMMARY

While theorists and researchers have yet to agree on a single, universally accepted theory or definition of spirituality, few would deny its existence or impact on health and healing. Recent research strongly points to the mind-body-spirit connection and to the essential relationship between the self, others, and a Higher Power or God. By caring for clients in a way that acknowledges this mind-body-spirit connection and by being present with their clients, health care providers acknowledge the whole person. By becoming familiar with the characteristics and essential elements of spirituality and utilizing this knowledge in caring for clients, health care providers become more than technicians—they move toward the role of healer.

KEY CONCEPTS

1. Spirituality is a multidimensional phenomenon that transcends gender, race, color, and national origin.
2. The centrality of the relationships between self, others, and God is one of the main focuses of spirituality and a prominent emerging theme in the literature.
3. A basic element of spirituality is meaning and purpose in life.
4. Spiritual development is individualistic and involves a series of steps or cycles that occur in no particular order or timeframe throughout the life of an individual.
5. The spiritual process of healing attends to the wholeness of an individual; occurs over time; is ongoing through one's life journey; and is a way of living that flows from, reflects, and nourishes one's spirit.

QUESTIONS FOR REFLECTION

1. How do you define spirituality and what does spirituality mean to you?
2. In what ways do you think spirituality affects health and healing? Do you believe in a mind-body-spirit connection? If not, what are some of the ways in which you can support clients who do?

REFERENCES

Bellingham, R., Cohen, B., Jones, T., & Spaniol, L. (1989). Connectedness: Some skills for spiritual health. *American Journal of Health Promotion, 24*(4), 18-24, 31.

Bergquist, S., & King, J. (1994). Parish nursing: A conceptual framework. *Journal of Holistic Nursing, 12*(2), 155-170.

Blazer, D. (1991). Spirituality and aging well. *Aging Well, 15*(1), 61-65.

Boudreaux, E. D., O'Hea, E., & Chasuk, R. (2002). Spiritual role in healing: An alternative way of thinking. *Primary Care: Clinics in Office Practice, 29*(2), 439-454.

Burkhardt, M. (1989). Spirituality: An analysis of the concept. *Holistic Nursing Practice, 3*(3), 69-77.

Burkhardt, M. A., & Nagai-Jacobson, M. G. (2002). *Spirituality: Living our connectedness.* New York: Delmar Thomson Learning.

Carson, V. B. (1989). *Spiritual dimensions of nursing practice.* Philadelphia: W.B. Saunders.

Chandler, E. (1999). Spirituality. *Hospice Journal, 14*(34), 63-74.

Chapman, L. S. (1987). Developing a useful perspective on spiritual health: Well-being, spiritual potential and the search for meaning. *American Journal of Health Promotion, 1*(3), 31-39.

Cobb, M., & Robshaw, V. (1998). *The spiritual challenge of health care.* New York: Churchill Livingstone.

Coyle, J. (2002). Spirituality and health: Towards a framework for exploring the relationship between spirituality and health. *Journal of Advanced Nursing, 37*(6), 589-597.

Dossey, B. M. (1997). *Core curriculum for holistic nursing.* Gaithersburg, MD: Aspen.

Dossey, B. M., Keegan, L., & Guzzetta, C. E. (2000). *Holistic nursing: A handbook for practice* (3rd ed.). Gaithersburg, MD: Aspen.

Dossey, L. (2001). *Healing beyond the body: Medicine and the infinite reach of the mind.* Boston: Shambhala.

Draper, P., & McSherry, W. (2002). A critical view of spirituality and spiritual assessment. *Journal of Advanced Nursing, 39*(1), 1-2.

Dyer, W. W. (2001). *There's a spiritual solution to every problem.* New York: HarperCollins.

Dyson, J., Cobb, M., & Forman, D. (1997). The meaning of spirituality: A literature review. *Journal of Advanced Nursing, 26*(6), 1183-1188.

Ebersole, P., & Hess, P. (1997). *Toward healthy aging: Human needs and nursing response* (5th ed.). St. Louis, MO: Mosby-Year Book.

Enblen, J. D. (1992). Religion and spirituality defined according to current use in nursing literature. *Journal of Professional Nursing, 8*(1), 41-47.

Falk-Rafael, A. R. (2000). Watson's philosophy, science, and theory of human caring as a conceptual framework for guiding community health nursing practice. *Advances in Nursing Practice, 23*(2), 34-49.

Fawcett, J. (2001). The nurse theorists: 21st-century updates: Betty Neuman. *Nursing Science Quarterly, 14*(3), 211-214.

Fehring, R. J., Miller, J. F., & Shaw, C. (1997). Spiritual well-being, religiosity, hope, depression, and other mood states in elderly people coping with cancer. *Oncology Nursing Forum, 24*(4), 663-671.

Fowler, J. (1987). *Faith development and pastoral care.* Philadelphia: Fortress Press.

Goddard, N. C. (2000). A response to Dawson's critical analysis of "spirituality" as "integrative energy." *Journal of Advanced Nursing, 31*(4), 968-979.

Goldberg, B. (1998). Connection: An exploration of spirituality in nursing care. *Journal of Advanced Nursing, 27*(4), 836-842.

Hasselkus, B. R. (2002). *The meaning of everyday occupation.* Thorofare, NJ: SLACK Incorporated.

Hatch, R. L., Burg, M. A., Naberhaus, D. S., & Hellmich, L. K. (1998). The spiritual involvement and beliefs scale: Development and testing of a new instrument. *Journal of Family Practice, 46*(6), 476-486.

Hiatt, J. F. (1986). Spirituality, medicine, and healing. *Southern Medical Journal, 79*(6), 736-743.

Hinds, P. (1988). Adolescent hopefulness in illness and health. *Advances in Nursing Science, 10*(3), 79-88.

Hungelmann, J., Kenkel-Rossi, E., Klassen, L., & Stollenwerk, R. M. (1985). Spiritual well-being in older adults: Harmonious interconnectedness. *Journal of Religion and Health, 24*(2), 147-153.

Isaia, D., Parker, V., & Murrow, E. (1999). Spiritual well-being among older adults. *Journal of Gerontological Nursing, 25*(8), 16-21.

Kleindienst, M. J. (1998). Spirituality: Where there is hope, there is life. *American Nephrology Nurses' Association, 25*(4), 442.

Knight, J. B. (1990). The Betty Neuman systems model applied to practice: A client with multiple sclerosis. *Journal of Advanced Nursing, 15*, 447-455.

Koenig, H. G., Idler, E., Kasl, S., Hays, J., George, L. K., Musick, M., et al. (1999). Religion, spirituality, and medicine: A rebuttal to skeptics. *International Journal of Psychiatry in Medicine, 29*(2), 123-131.

Larson, D. B., Swyers, J. P., & McCullough, M. E. (1998). *Scientific research on spirituality and health.* Rockville, MD: National Institute for Healthcare Research.

Leetun, M. C. (1996). Wellness and spirituality in the older adult: Assessment and intervention protocol. *Nurse Practitioner, 21*(8), 60, 65-70.

Macrae, J. A. (2001). *Nursing as a spiritual practice: A contemporary application of Florence Nightingale's views.* New York: Springer.

Mahoney, M. J., & Graci, G. M. (1999). The meanings and correlates of spirituality: Suggestions from an exploratory survey of experts. *Death Studies, 23*(6), 521-529.

Mansen, T. J. (1993). The spiritual dimension of individuals: Conceptual development. *Nursing Diagnosis, 4*(4), 140-146.

Martsolf, D. S., & Mickley, J. R. (1998). The concept of spirituality in nursing theories: Differing world-views and extent of focus. *Journal of Advanced Nursing, 27*(2), 294-303.

McSherry, W., & Draper, P. (1998). The debates emerging from the literature surrounding the concept of spirituality as applied to nursing. *Journal of Advanced Nursing, 27*(4), 683-691.

Meraviglia, M. G. (1999). Critical analysis of spirituality and its empirical indicators. *Journal of Holistic Nursing, 17*(1), 18-33.

Messikomer, C., & De Craemer, W. (2002). The spirituality of academic physicians: An ethnography of a scripture-based group in an academic medical center. *Academic Medicine, 77*(6), 562-573.

Miller, M. (1995). Culture, spirituality, and women's health. *JOGNN Clinical Issues, 24*(3), 257-263.

Miller, W. R. (Ed.). (1999). *Integrating spirituality into treatment: Resources for practitioners.* Washington, DC: American Psychological Association.

Moran, M. (1999). What is the role of spirituality in medicine? *American Medical News, 42*(14), 1-3.

Narayanasamy, A. (1999). A review of spirituality as applied to nursing. *International Journal of Nursing Studies, 36*, 117-125.

Owen, D. (1989). Nurses' perspectives on the meaning of hope in patients with cancer: A qualitative study. *Oncology Nurses Forum, 16*, 75-79.

Parse, R. R. (1992). Human becoming: Parse's theory of nursing. *Nursing Science Quarterly, 5*(1), 35-42.

Pilch, J. J. (1988). Wellness spirituality. *Health Values, 12*(3), 28-31.

Reynolds, C. (2001). *Spiritual fitness.* London: Thorsons.

Saewyc, E. M. (2000). Nursing theories of caring: A paradigm for adolescent nursing practice. *Journal of Holistic Nursing, 18*(2), 114-128.

Shea, J. (2000). *Spirituality and health care.* Chicago: Park Ridge Center for the Study of Health, Faith, and Ethics.

Skokan, L., & Bader, D. (2000). Spirituality and healing. *Health Progress, 81*(1), 1-8.

Spaniol, L. (2002). Spirituality and connectedness. *Psychiatric Rehabilitation Journal, 25*(2), 321-322.

Streeter, C. M. (1996). What is spirituality? *Health Progress, 77*(3), 17-22.

Taylor, E. J. (2002). *Spiritual care.* Upper Saddle River, NJ: Prentice Hall.

Thomason, C. L., & Brody, H. (1999). Inclusive spirituality. *Journal of Family Practice, 48*(2), 96-97.

Tuck, I., Wallace, D., & Pullen, L. (2001). Spirituality and spiritual care provided by parish nurses. *Western Journal of Nursing Research, 23*(5), 441-453.

Walton, J. (1996). Spiritual relationships: A concept analysis. *Journal of Holistic Nursing, 14*(3), 237-250.

Walton, J. (1999). Spirituality of patients recovering from an acute myocardial infarction. *Journal of Holistic Nursing, 17*(1), 34-53.

Watson, M. J. (1988). New dimensions of human caring theory. *Nursing Science Quarterly, 1*(4), 175-181.

Weil, A. (1997). *Eight weeks to optimum health.* New York: Alfred A. Knopf.

Zerwekh, J. (1997). The practice of presencing. *Seminars in Oncology Nursing, 13*(4), 260-262.

2

SPIRITUALITY, THE HEALTH CARE PROFESSIONAL, AND THE SPIRITUAL CARE PROVIDER

"Make us, Lord, worthy to serve our brothers and sisters who are scattered all over the world, who live and die alone and poor. Give them today, using our hands, their daily bread. And, using our love, give them peace and happiness. Amen."
—Mother Teresa

LEARNING OBJECTIVES

Upon completing this chapter, you will be able to do the following:
1. Describe the relationship between health care providers, spirituality, and religion.
2. Identify the types of spiritual care generalists and specialists and describe their role in providing spiritual care.
3. Describe the influence of a health care provider's spirituality on his or her ability to provide spiritual care.
4. List barriers to providing spiritual care to clients.
5. Explain key moral and ethical considerations when providing spiritual care.

INTRODUCTION

The spiritual relationship that occurs between health care provider and client can provide both parties with a sense of strength, inner peace, healing, harmonious interconnectedness, and meaning (Walton, 1996). By caring, listening, and engendering trust, the health care provider and the client can form a spiritual relationship that can heal each other. The provision of care and the illness experience can be deeply personal experiences that cause fundamental questions of "why" and "how" to be raised. "Why me?" and "How do I view my relationship with a Higher

Power?" are just some of the questions that lead the care provider (as well as the client) to examine the experiences of pain, suffering, life and death, and injustice. Yet why is this spiritual relationship often difficult to achieve?

Perhaps it is because Western medicine, in which many health care providers have been indoctrinated, has tended to define health as the absence of disease and to reduce the human body to distinct parts that must be "fixed" if the individual is to function optimally. This type of care supports a belief in the real and the observable and looks at the individual as a compilation of parts. Nonrational, nontraditional aspects of health and illness are often overlooked or even dismissed as unscientific, unreliable, and therefore invalid (Messikomer & De Craemer, 2002). The Western model of medicine has helped those in health care remain objective and "face the unknown without disruptive emotional reactivity" (Hiatt, 1986, p. 742). This perspective, however, may contribute significantly to the dissatisfaction with health care experienced by many individuals and health care practitioners alike. It may also adversely affect the way in which care is delivered (Hiatt, 1986).

The connection between spirituality and health care may not seem obvious to some, since health care and the scientific knowledge that forms its foundation have, for centuries, existed separately from religion. Yet nursing and medicine, in particular, have their very origins in religion and spirituality. Nurses have been called "angels of mercy," and many health care providers believe their work is a "calling" with unique requirements, responsibilities, and distinct moral duties. Health care providers witness human dramas that cause existential questions to be raised. In no other field can an individual witness and participate in critical, life-threatening, life-renewing, or life-sustaining experiences on a day-to-day basis. Spirituality becomes almost tangible when individuals face crises, emotional stress, physical illness, or death and is often the very force that provides health care providers with the strength to face the daily challenges of their profession.

Health care organizations are now obligated to respond to the spiritual needs of their clients because clients have a right to holistic care that addresses their physical, emotional, and spiritual needs. For example, the Joint Commission on the Accreditation of Healthcare Organizations (JCAHO) and the Canadian Council on Health Services Accreditation both have statements requiring health care teams to consider the client's spiritual values and needs in the delivery of care. As a result, most health care organizations have clients' rights statements that pledge to provide care supporting the "dignity, culture, beliefs, practices, and spiritual needs of all patients, their caregivers, and hospital personnel" (VandeCreek & Burton, 2001, p. 3).

Spirituality is a part of every human condition and an intimate part of health and illness. Caring for the "whole" person requires a close relationship between spirituality, the health care provider, and the spiritual care provider. The health care provider's own spirituality has a powerful impact on his or her ability to provide spiritual care, as do a number of other barriers that can arise. In addition, moral and ethical considerations also come into play when providing spiritual care. This chapter will explore each of these elements in detail.

SPIRITUAL HEALTH CARE PROVIDERS

Spiritual care can be provided by many different individuals. In one study, clients with cancer ranked their preference for resource persons. In descending order, they listed family and friends, personal clergy, physicians, nurses, chaplains, psychiatrists or psychologists, and social workers (Taylor, 2002).

When providing spiritual care to a client, health care providers have numerous resources upon which to draw. According to Taylor (2002), nurses, physicians, and social workers are *spiritual care generalists*, while chaplains, clergy, parish nurses, spiritual mentors, family and friends, and folk healers are considered *spiritual care specialists*. Each type will be briefly described.

Spiritual Care Generalists

Health care professionals who provide various types of care, including spiritual care, are described as spiritual care generalists.

Nurses

Modern-day nursing has its beginnings with the efforts of Florence Nightingale, whose view of nursing was derived from a profound spiritual philosophy. She believed spirituality was an essential part of human nature and the most potent resource for healing (Louis & Alpert, 2000). Although she was not interested in traditional religion, Nightingale was interested in the writings of Western mystics such as St. Francis of Assisi and St. John of the Cross, as well as the Eastern scriptures. Rather than being at odds with spirituality, she believed science was the basis for a relationship with God (Macrae, 1995). Nightingale believed that the focus of nursing was to create an environment in which natural healing might take place. This environment included cleanliness, fresh air, sunlight, warmth, quiet, and proper nutrition (Dossey, Keegan, & Guzzetta, 2000). Nightingale believed that human beings needed to be considered from a physical, psychological, environmental, and spiritual perspective (Bergquist & King, 1994).

Historically, the profession of nursing has strong links and affiliations with religious and spiritual traditions, especially Christianity. In this context, nursing is a manifestation of God's love expressed through caring, compassion, and charity toward the sick and the poor (McSherry & Draper, 1998). Nursing saw the patient as a "whole" and treated him or her holistically. Nightingale was an advocate of holistic care and did not treat the patient as simply a disease. She recognized a force that healed and was greater than herself (Dossey, 2000).

During the last half of the 20th century, sophisticated technologies and "hard" sciences began to overshadow the importance of spirituality in nursing care. Nursing as a profession became more complex, and the relevance of spirituality began to fade (McSherry & Draper, 1998). For example, nursing curricula during the 1960s and 1970s emphasized chemistry, anatomy, physiology, microbiology, and pathophysiology rather than the spiritual aspects of care (Louis & Alpert, 2000). As a profession, nursing strived to be taken more seriously and so focused on the scientific method as well as the tangible, materialistic aspects of human nature and physiology. Nursing, comprised mostly of women, followed the lead of mainstream society and the biological, reductionist approach to health care. Thus, nurses became increasingly subordinate to physicians, who were mostly male (McSherry & Draper, 1998). As technology became more sophisticated, tasks that were once the exclusive domain of nursing were no longer relevant, and nursing had to re-examine its role in the provision of care (Martsolf & Mickley, 1998).

Many nurses consider themselves to be religious, and many consider their own personal religious training to be adequate training for spiritual caregiving. In reality, this misconception may influence the practice of many nurses and result in the provision of inadequate spiritual care. Many nurses have had no formal education in spiritual care skills except for some basic information received during training. However, more and more nurses are acquiring education in this area through various informal and formal programs, chaplaincy training, or graduate programs in pastoral counseling or ministry. Trained nurses can provide excellent spiritual care and can also appropriately refer clients to other spiritual care providers.

Physicians

The physician-client relationship, like that of other health care providers with their clients, is essentially a spiritual relationship (Boudreaux, O'Hea, & Chasuk, 2002). Many clients wish their physicians would talk to them about spiritual matters, pray with them, or draw on spiritual coping resources during times of crisis (Larson & Koenig, 2000; Miller, 1999).

During one survey at a meeting of the American Academy of Family Physicians, 99% of physicians stated they believed religious beliefs can heal and 75% believed that the prayers of others can aid in healing. Yet, most of these physicians also reported that they rarely discussed spiritual issues with their clients (Larimore, 2001; O'Hara, 2002). In one study, only 10% of physicians discussed spiritual issues with their clients, even though the majority of clients stated that they would like to have their physicians discuss spiritual matters with them (Larson & Koenig, 2000).

Religion is often considered the antithesis of modern medical care; thus, many physicians consider it inappropriate and even unethical to discuss religion and spiritual matters with their clients (Larimore, 2001; Larson & Koenig, 2000). Many physicians have not received training in the area of spiritual care, and they may not make referrals to the appropriate spiritual care provider. Others state they do not feel comfortable taking a spiritual history, some do not know how to identify clients who want to discuss spiritual issues, and others do not know how to manage spiritual issues once they are raised (Larimore, 2001).

Some health care providers recommend that physicians should not attempt to address complex spiritual needs of clients unless they have received some education in this area and fully understand the relationship between religion, spirituality, and health; otherwise, they may be perceived as potentially coercive (Koenig, 2001). However, as more and more physicians receive training in this area and study the results of research on the importance of spirituality in health, they will assume a more active role in the spiritual care process.

Social Workers

The social worker plays an important part in bridging the gap between physical and psychosocial care of the patient and family. The social worker, in conjunction with other members of the team, works to identify the patient and family experience of suffering, and then develops strategies to ease it. (Kuebler, Berry, & Heidrich, 2002, p. 10)

Social workers may assist in the spiritual care process in many ways, including helping families organize their care support system and guiding the client and family in meeting their emotional, spiritual, psychological, and bereavement needs.

Spiritual Care Specialists

When specific interventions are needed, spiritual care generalists often refer clients to spiritual care specialists—those with specific training and formal education in areas such as spiritual care, pastoral counseling, theology, and psychology.

Chaplains

Chaplains are professionals who represent "a merger of theology and psychology" (Taylor, 2002, p. 181). An estimated 9,000 chaplains in the United States help people with health-related transitions (Taylor, 2002).

Where Can Chaplains Be Found?

Chaplains provide spiritual care in many types of health care settings, including the following:

- Acute care
- Long-term care
- Assisted living
- Rehabilitation
- Mental health
- Outpatient units
- Addiction treatment facilities
- Hospice and palliative care

Chaplains are professionally accountable to their religious faith group, their certifying chaplaincy organization, and their employing institution. They can provide spiritual care to all types of individuals, including actively religious persons who may not notify their religious community leaders of their hospitalization, other hospitalized or ill individuals who do not belong to a religious or spiritual community, and individuals who may be far from their spiritual leader when they become ill (VandeCreek & Burton, 2001).

JCAHO requires that institutions make formal arrangements for chaplain services (Taylor, 2002; VandeCreek & Burton, 2001). Some institutions use professional chaplains while others use volunteer chaplains.

Professional chaplains can obtain their certification from several sources. They must possess a graduate degree in theology or ministry, be recognized as clergy members by their religious denomination, and be endorsed by a faith group for ministry as chaplains. In addition, they can become certified by completing a specific number of clinical hours of clinical pastoral education (CPE) from the Association for Clinical Pastoral Education (ACPE), the United States Catholic Conference/National Association of Catholic Chaplains (NACC), or the Canadian Association for Pastoral Practice and Education (CAPPE). A minimum of 1 year of additional training or residency as a chaplain is required to complete the certification (Association of Professional Chaplains, 2002). Chaplains are also required to pass written and oral examinations before becoming certified by the Association of Professional Chaplains (Koenig, 2000).

In *Spiritual Care: Nursing Theory, Research, and Practice*, Taylor (2002) describes four broad roles that pertain to chaplains:

- Conducting spiritual assessments.
- Responding to clients' religious concerns and helping them with religious coping strategies.
- Supporting professional staff.
- Functioning as a liaison with religious communities (e.g., nurses consult with chaplains for many reasons, including helping with family support in times of death, emergencies, or difficult decision making; arranging bedside religious rites; helping with cessation of life support; or assisting with an anxious or fearful client).

Chaplains frequently function as members of one or more treatment teams where they act as interpreters to the staff about religious or spiritual issues related to clients. In addition, they can also provide the following services (VandeCreek & Burton, 2001):

- Educate the health care team as well as the community about how multifaith and multicultural traditions can impact clinical services.
- Provide community educational topics on spirituality, loss and illness, and coping with crisis.
- Clarify institutional policies to clients, clergy, and religious organizations.
- Serve as contact persons for arranging the assessment for the appropriateness and coordination of complementary therapies.
- Protect clients from being confronted by unwelcome forms of spiritual intrusion, such as proselytizing.
- Serve as members of health care ethics programs.
- Help clients and their families identify their values regarding end-of-life care.
- Improve communication between staff and families, thus reducing expensive, unwanted care.
- Assist staff in coping with their own grief and provide education in the areas of ethics, spirituality, or coping strategies, thus freeing the staff to attend to other duties.

Clergy

For many people, the first person they seek out during times of crisis and need is their pastor, rabbi, or priest. This individual may already know the individual on a personal level and be particularly helpful in working with that individual to understand the available spiritual support and health care resources (Miller, 1999). Many persons would rather seek help from their clergy than from mental health professionals and are often more satisfied with the assistance they receive from clergy (Koenig, 2000). Others may not contact their clergy because they may be embarrassed about the circumstances surrounding their care or believe their situation does not necessitate contact with a clergy member (Taylor, 2002).

Counseling by community clergy is often free of charge and does not carry the stigma that a visit to a psychologist or psychiatrist might carry (Koenig, 2000). Clergy are professionals who have been trained in the religious ministry, but their training can be highly variable. While some have little or no college education, others have earned master's degrees. Some may not have received any training in how to help clients through health care crises, while others may be highly qualified to assist in this area (Taylor, 2002). Many have not received training in mental health counseling and may not recognize when a person needs professional assistance (Koenig, 2000). Per specific institutional policy, chaplains often make referrals to clergy, and nurses need to be sensitive to this practice. However, in other organizations, nurses can initiate referrals.

Because many clergy have clinical pastoral education as part of their training, clergy often work with a client's therapist to help him or her better understand the client as well as the spiritual assistance available through that client's spiritual community (Miller, 1999).

Parish Nurses

Parish nurses have their roots in ancient civilizations with the integration of religion and health. During the development of scientific thought, however, spirituality and healing were separated. Today, with the renewed interest in holistic care, parish nursing is growing tremendously. Reverend Granger Westberg, a doctor of divinity from Chicago, founded the current parish nursing movement in the mid-1980s, and there are currently thousands of parish nurses practicing in almost every state in the United States as well as all over the world. Parish nursing is now considered a specialty by the American Nurses Association (ANA); as such, parish nursing has established standards and a clearly defined scope of practice (Bergquist & King, 1994; Ebersole, 2000).

A parish nurse is an experienced registered nurse with specialized training in holistic health and spiritual care. He or she has "spiritual maturity and a commitment to healing ministries" (Tuck, Wallace, & Pullen, 2001, p. 442). While their educational background may vary, most parish nurses receive their training in spiritual caregiving; philosophy, health assessment, and psychosocial issues; community resources; and the professional, legal, and ethical issues that are specific to their role (Ebersole, 2000). Referral to a parish nurse is especially relevant when the client's health concerns relate to his or her religious practices.

By grouping individuals according to congregation or religious affiliation, parish nursing strives to identify populations by means of "their value orientation, spiritual direction, and community and cultural associations" (Hitchcock, Schubert, & Thomas, 1999, p. 329). Parish nurses provide holistic care to members of a specific religious congregation and they know their parishioners intimately. Parish nurses collaborate with the clergy and parish staff and strive to promote health and prevent disease. They also act as the following:

- Integrators of faith and health
- Health educators
- Role models
- Personal health counselors
- Volunteer coordinators
- Advocates and facilitators
- Support group developers
- Referral agents or community liaisons
- Interpreters of the relationship between faith and health (Boland, 1998; Louis & Alpert, 2000; Tuck et al., 2001)

The expertise of parish nurses expands the services unique to home care or public health nurses. Parish nurses do not perform hands-on, invasive procedures or administer medications (Bergquist & King, 1994; Tuck et al., 2001). They do provide a framework to help individuals and families move toward healthier states (Hitchcock et al., 1999).

Parish nurses may practice under one of four types of models (Bergquist & King, 1994):

1. **The institutional/paid model:** A paid parish nurse is an employee for an institution such as a hospital, agency, or long-term care facility.
2. **The institutional/volunteer model:** Services are provided by a nurse in the faith community interested in volunteering his or her time with the institution providing resources, continuing education classes, and/or supervision.
3. **The congregation/paid model:** The parish nurse is employed by the faith community or ministerial association to provide services to one or more faith communities.
4. **The congregational/volunteer model:** The parish nurse receives no money or stipend, and the resources required may be purchased by the congregation, local community agencies, or an external network of parish nurses.

Spiritual Mentors

These individuals are "spiritual directors" who help others develop spiritually. They can be of any religious denomination and they often meet regularly with their clients to work on spiritual goals or spiritual issues. They may have received special training and may be religious professionals. They can provide encouragement and comfort, as well as challenge individuals to increase their spiritual awareness and discipline (Taylor, 2002).

Family and Friends

These individuals may or may not have spiritual training, but clients often indicate they are needed when the clients require spiritual nurturing. Family and friends can function as supportive companions by providing assistance with prayer, reading, or singing; providing comforting thoughts; sharing a healing ritual; or providing much-needed empathy. Because friends and family share an intimate history with the client, they can provide a type of support that no other individuals can provide (Taylor, 2002).

Folk Healers

In many cultures, health and spirituality are intimately interwoven, and the healing of physical and mental illness is sought from individuals who are believed to have special healing abilities. Folk healing systems are "a formal, coherent, and consistent set of beliefs and practices ascribed to a particular culture" (Wing, 1999, p. 257). Beliefs and practices are usually part of an oral tradition in which knowledge is passed from one generation to another after healers complete a specific selection process and education (a calling, apprenticeship, or schooling) (Wing, 1999). At the beginning of the 20th century in the United States, alternative and folk healers were the exception rather than the rule. As Western medicine grew, these healers were used less and less. Now, with the resurgence of interest in complementary and alternative medicine, many people are seeking a simpler way of addressing life events that can affect health (Huch, 1999).

These folk or lay healers focus on a holistic framework of health and well-being that promotes harmony rather than diagnosis and curing. Examples of folk and lay healers include the Native American medicine men, Mexican curanderos, and "neighborhood women" (a form of folk healers in the Hispanic community). They use techniques unique to their culture and usually quite different from traditional Western medicine. Folk healers often have specific attributes and a defined status within their culture. They may use special rituals, herbs, or other natural materials to promote health, and they usually receive their education as the result of an apprenticeship, personal study, or experience (Bonder, Martin, & Miracle, 2002; Engebretson, 1996; Taylor, 2002).

Folk healers may be used instead of or in conjunction with Western biomedical practitioners. Those who turn to curanderos, for example, believe their cultural practices are justified because they deal routinely with social, psychological, physical, and/or spiritual issues that are often ignored by conventional physicians (Trotter, 2001). Some believe that certain folk healing beliefs and practices, such as healing, holism, and therapeutic touch, are the "very essence of contemporary nursing" (Wing, 1999, p. 256).

The use of local remedies is only one aspect of folk healing. Another equally important aspect is the meaning assigned to sickness and the beliefs and acts associated with the special ministrations (Zapata & Shippee-Rice, 1999). The cultures that use folk healers often consider sickness the result of a sin; God's punishment; causal agents such as lightning, water, or wind (Navajo Indians); negative thoughts or pathogens (Cherokee); or evil spirits. Therefore, folk healing focuses on the use of magical powers, special gifts, and rituals to restore balance (Cohen, 1998; Milne & Howard, 2000; Zapata & Shippee-Rice, 1999).

Shamans, for example, are specialized healers who "mix practical remedies and advice with abstractions, often couched in stories, songs, and dance" (Bonder et al., 2002, p. 30). They possess the role of physician and priest and act as "a guide to the soul" (Rhi, 2001, p. 569). A widely practiced curing ritual of Andean shamans in South America is to suck the foreign spirits or matter from a sick individual. During the process, the individual's family members concentrate their healing energies on the process to increase the power of the shaman to heal the individual. In this way, all those affected by the illness help facilitate the healing (Bonder et al., 2002).

Athabascan Shamans

The Athabascan Indians along the Yukon River believed that:
> ...people become sick because a spirit called the Giyeg thought about them—just as though he was setting a trap for them. If a person was captured by this spirit and nothing was done to distract him, the victim would die in one or two days. (Carroll, 2002, p. 67)

Athabascan shamans guard people against the effects of evil spirits, diagnose various maladies, and restore to health those who have been harmed by evil spirits by recapturing the spirit (utilizing the special contents of a medicine bag) and removing foreign objects. White men are believed to be inhabited by the soul of a deceased Indian and are, therefore, considered ghosts with no soul, so the power of the Athabascan shaman is ineffective in dealing with the white man (Carroll, 2002).

Folk healers may utilize many types of activities to support their client on the journey to total well-being. These include the following (Engebretson, 1996; Milne & Howard, 2000; Wing, 1999):

- Affirmations
- Visualizations
- A positive attitude
- Relaxation and stress-reduction techniques
- Healing energy
- Supporting positive relationships in the client's life
- Encouraging time in nature
- Meditation
- Visual arts to represent the Holy People in their human form (Navajo sand-paintings)
- Music
- Healing ceremonies
- Connecting with God or a Higher Power
- Faith, prayer, and hope

According to Zapata & Shippee-Rice (1999), folk healers—especially curanderos—often conceal their identity to members of the "outside" culture as well as to members of their own culture because of a fear of punishment from both the legal and health care community.

THE SPIRITUALITY OF HEALTH CARE PROVIDERS

While health care providers may describe themselves as religious or spiritual, many lack the formal education that could prepare them to administer effective spiritual care. In addition, they may not know where to obtain that education or where to enhance the education and information they already possess. This lack of education may cause them to be uncomfortable when assessing their clients and providing spiritual care.

One way for providers to effectively begin their spiritual education is to conduct a personal inventory of their own spirituality. Examining their belief system, their commitment to spiritual care in health care, their strengths for providing spiritual care, and their needs for further personal development in the role of spiritual caregiver can be an important first step toward providing spiritual care. (Additional tools for self-assessment will be covered in Chapters 5 and 6.) The following questions can be used as a guide in this personal inventory (Dossey et al., 2000, pp. 106-108):

- Is faith important to me?
- Do I believe in God or a Higher Power?
- Do I participate in religious activities?
- Do I pray?
- Do I believe spiritual care is an important component in providing health care?
- What strengths do I have to offer as a spiritual care provider?
- What areas do I need to strengthen in order to provide sensitive, compassionate spiritual care to my clients?

Providing spiritual care involves not only *doing* spiritual activities but also *being* spiritual (Dossey et al., 2000). Being spiritual means developing characteristics that influence the ability to be an instrument of healing. These characteristics can include the following (Taylor, 2002):

- Appreciation of self-healing as a constant process
- Openness to self-discovery
- Clarity of life's purpose
- Awareness of areas for personal growth so insight can be gained and shared
- Self-nurturing and the ability to model that self-care for clients
- A perspective that recognizes that time with clients is an opportunity for sharing and serving

Self-awareness requires health care professionals to identify and address their feelings. Anger, jealousy, grief, and fear all have a purpose. For example, fear can help people be more cautious. To manage feelings in a healthy way, health care professionals need to have "safe" people with whom to talk and "safe" situations in which to talk about and learn from their feelings (Taylor, 2002).

Taylor (2002) states that "spirituality is not separate from daily life" (p. 64). Health care professionals can cultivate their spiritual self-awareness by finding spirituality at work or in their daily life. Taking the time to have a prayer experience while sitting in traffic or taking advantage of quiet moments to be still are some methods for cultivating spirituality.

Health care professionals are involved in spiritual care just by the nature of the care they provide. Care given in a loving, compassionate, warm, and generous manner provides clients with a safe place to "surrender, to establish new intimacies, and to become the person whom they choose to be" (Leetun, 1996, p. 69). When health care professionals can accept their own vulnerability, they see the vulnerability in others and this strengthens their relationship to their clients (Leetun, 1996).

BARRIERS TO PROVIDING SPIRITUAL CARE

While many health care providers agree that there is a link between spirituality and health, many are reluctant to develop and use the skills needed to assess a client's spiritual beliefs and needs and to deliver spiritual care. One study suggested that up to 77% of clients would like spiritual issues considered as part of their overall health care (Anandarajah & Hight, 2001). In another study, 53% of oncology nurses rarely or never prayed with their clients, 66% rarely or never read religious or spiritual passages with a client, and the majority rarely or never addressed the client's relationship with a Higher Power (Davidhizar, Bechtel, & Juratovac, 2000).

There are many reasons for this reluctance. Some health care providers lack an education in spiritual caregiving and thus lack confidence in their ability to provide spiritual care. Others lack the time necessary for the assessment; they cite the short length of stay in the hospital, the presence of environmental distractions resulting in loss of privacy, fear of invading a client's privacy, worry about the inappropriateness of addressing spiritual needs, or lack of personal spiritual awareness (Brush & Daly, 2000; Burkhardt & Nagai-Jacobson, 2002; Davidhizar et al., 2000; Hodge, 2001; Hurley, 1999; Louis & Alpert, 2000; McSherry & Cash, 2000; O'Connor, 2001; Wright, 1998, 2002).

Still others believe that spirituality is synonymous with religion, and they feel that spiritual care requires a mastery of the beliefs of each religious tradition. Health care providers may also feel that to ask a client about spirituality is a thinly disguised way of proselytizing about their own particular faith beliefs (Louis & Alpert, 2000; Thomason & Brody, 1990). Many health care providers also believe that spiritual assessment lies solely within the realm of spiritual experts, such as chaplains (Wright, 2002).

Spiritual care involves the intangible, difficult-to-measure features of an individual that "contrast sharply with the contemporary focus on high-tech, physical care" of today's health care environment (Wright, 2002, p. 129). Physicians are often reluctant to explore spiritual issues because of the perceived lack of a tested, reliable method for assessing spirituality (Hatch, Burg, Naberhaus, & Hellmich, 1998).

The nursing profession has fought long and hard for respect as a profession whose practice and therapies are based on scientific principles. As a result, nurses may feel uncomfortable discussing spiritual issues with a client, since the spiritual dimension is still so difficult to define and measure. Nurses may have difficulty separating their clients' spiritual dimension from their psychosocial dimension. This failure to distinguish between the two has led to spiritual problems being diagnosed and treated as psychosocial problems (Mansen, 1993). However, most contemporary nursing models recognize the importance of a holistic approach to client care. The spiritual attitudes of life, including love, joy, kindness, goodness, faithfulness, self-control, hope, gentleness, and patience, do not cease to exist because an individual becomes a client. As Kleindienst (1998) writes, "Patients without hope are usually in more need of meaning than medication" (p. 442).

Clients may also present barriers to the provision of spiritual care. These can include their fears of being misjudged, their lack of knowledge about spirituality and its impact on health, their inability to communicate because of an illness or loss of senses, or their own prejudices about their care providers (McSherry & Cash, 2000).

Other barriers that can be present on the part of the client or the provider include "dehumanizing" behaviors such as directive, degrading, judgmental, monological, careless behaviors that isolate and control the other individual (Walton, 1996).

Regardless of these barriers, the health care provider has a professional responsibility to assess a client's spiritual needs (O'Connor, 2001). Barriers to providing spiritual care can be overcome in many ways. Taking responsibility for providing competent spiritual care is the first step. This can be achieved through a deeper understanding of the health care provider's own spiritual dimension, as well as reading, self-study, and involvement in workshops and education on spirituality and healing (Burkhardt & Nagai-Jacobson, 2002).

In addition, it is important to realize that performing spiritual assessments and providing spiritual care does not require the health care professional to solve all of his or her clients' problems or accept responsibility for their choices. It can simply mean listening to them and letting them share their own stories. Spiritual care also does not mean imposing one's spiritual values on others. People who are clear about their own spiritual beliefs are less likely to impose their values and beliefs on others and, instead, appreciate their own traditions while understanding the spiritual expressions of others (Burkhardt & Nagai-Jacobson, 2002).

MORAL AND ETHICAL ISSUES IN SPIRITUAL CARE

Morality, ethics, and spirituality are inextricably related and intertwined with culture, religion, values, emotions, and the social aspects of an individual (Taylor, 2002). Health care professionals "find their origin, purpose, and meaning within the context of culturally accepted moral norms, individual values, and perceived social need" (Burkhardt & Nathaniel, 1998, p. 3).

- **Morality** deals with what is "good" or "bad," "right" or "wrong." It "investigates moral duties, values, and ideal human character" (Salladay & McDonnell, 1989, p. 543). According to Taylor (2002), morality refers to the "rules a society has created for promoting ethical conduct, or right and virtuous behavior" (p. 13).
- **Ethics** is concerned with what one "ought" or "should" do in any given situation, and it is the process by which morality is practiced (Burkhardt & Nathaniel, 1998). For example, a religion may consider something "wrong" to do, but society at large may consider it the "right" thing to do. The belief of a Jehovah Witness that blood transfusions are "wrong" can create an ethical dilemma, as well as an emotional one, when a health care provider believes it is the medically "right" thing to do to save the individual's life. Yet, the courts have consistently upheld the refusals of blood transfusions by competent adult Jehovah's Witnesses (Lo, 2000).
- **Values** contain potent emotional and spiritual significance and are powerful motivators of behavior. Ethical questions such as, "What is the right thing for me to do?" raise spiritual questions such as, "What is of value to me?" (Salladay & McDonnell, 1989).

If health care professionals truly believe in the holistic concept of client care, they have an ethical obligation to provide spiritual care (Davidhizar et al., 2000; Treloar, 2001; Wright, 1998). The words *health*, *holy*, and *whole* are derived from the old Saxon word *hal* and the Greek *holos*, which mean "whole" (McSherry & Cash, 2000). Thus, "by their nature, then, health and healing are associated with that which is holy and whole" (Burkhardt & Nathaniel, 1998, p. 327). The minimizing of this aspect of care or its neglect may have serious implications for the client's health or illness (O'Brien, 1999).

Ethical Principles

The major ethical principles of beneficence, nonmaleficence, autonomy, confidentiality, and advocacy apply to the spiritual care of clients. They may be helpful in assisting health care professionals when they encounter such questions as the following (DeLashmutt & Silva, 1998; Treloar, 2001):

- What should I do if the client or family invites me to pray with them?
- How can I give spiritual care without unduly influencing the client or the family?
- Can I give spiritual care if a client or family is of a different faith or religion than I?
- Should I initiate prayer for a client or family?
- Is it unethical to pray for a client without his or her consent?

Beneficence (i.e., the duty to do the right thing) obligates the health care provider to act in a positive way to benefit the client. This results in a level of trust between the provider and the client so the health care provider acts in such a way that the client will be helped and not harmed (Burkhardt & Nathaniel, 1998; Wright, 1998). An example of beneficence is the acknowledgement and support of a client's spirituality (Mueller, Plevak, & Rummans, 2001).

Nonmaleficence (i.e., the duty to do no harm to a client) is related to beneficence and means that a health care provider ought not act in such a way that could result in deliberate harm, risk of harm, or harm as a result of a beneficial act (Burkhardt & Nathaniel, 1998). It can be interpreted to mean that a health care professional must provide spiritual care as part of the overall care, since withholding spiritual care can negatively impact the client, and clients regard their spiritual health and physical health as equally important (Mueller et al., 2001).

Autonomy in relation to spiritual care can be interpreted to mean assisting clients with their spiritual needs without imposing one's own beliefs on that client. Autonomy means "self-governing" or "self-determination" and, when related to health care, means the individual has the freedom to make choices about his or her own life (Burkhardt & Nathaniel, 1998; Purtillo, 1999). People want the ability to make choices about their lives because the stakes associated with decision making can be high in health care (Lo, 2000). Autonomy is closely related to the concept of informed consent.

Confidentiality is the ethical principle that requires individuals who are entrusted with private or secret information to keep that information private or secret. Confidentiality is mentioned in the Nightingale Pledge for graduating nurses: "I will do all in my power to elevate the standard of my profession and will hold in confidence all personal matters committed to my keeping and all family affairs coming to my knowledge in the practice of my profession" (Thomas, 1997, p. 1301).

Confidentiality is also mentioned in the Hippocratic oath for physicians:

> Whatever, in connection with my professional practice, or not in connection with it, I see or hear, in the life of men, which out not to be spoken of abroad, I will not divulge, as reckoning that all such should be kept secret. (Thomas, 1997, p. 902)

While clergy, physicians, and lawyers have a professional-client privilege, nurse-client interactions are not considered legally privileged in most states in the United Sates (Wright, 1998).

Finally, *advocacy* involves helping clients exercise their autonomy. Health care professionals should always act in a way that promotes and safeguards the interests and well-being of their clients (McSherry & Cash, 2000). Advocacy requires the health care professional to "honor the dignity and freedom of the patient in a covenant relationship as modeled between God and believers" (Salladay & McDonnell, 1989, p. 543). The spiritual care provider who is a client advocate is able to set aside his or her personal agendas and help clients search for their own meaning during times of suffering, frustration, and vulnerability (Salladay & McDonnell, 1989).

Spiritual Care: An Ethical Obligation

Not everyone has spiritual needs that require attention all the time, and not all clients will require help from a health care professional about their spiritual needs. Many individuals are self-sufficient or have a variety of appropriate resources on which they may depend to help them with spiritual concerns (McSherry & Ross, 2002). Others, such as nonbelievers, may still be in need of spiritual care but the health care professional must be sensitive as to how to deliver this care and include clients in discussions about how best to meet their needs (McSherry & Cash, 2000). Others believe that, since spirituality cannot be measured, it might not be ethical to assist clients with their spiritual needs when health care providers cannot measure the impact of that intervention. Further, they believe that prescribing specific religious activities can be considered unethical and coercive since the relationship between client and provider is unequal. However, according to Treloar (2001), the relationship with God must be nurtured and expressed. Properly trained, spiritually aware health care and spiritual care professionals should be prepared to offer appropriate and ethical care that does not involve coercion and is more substantive than just prescribing religious activities.

Spirituality is an important part of wellness and an indispensable part of holistic care. Therefore, professional and ethical obligations oblige health care providers to develop their skills in the delivery of spiritual care.

SUMMARY

While many types of professionals can provide spiritual care, all people have the ability to heal themselves and be sacred healers (Shealey, 1999). Working together, the health care or spiritual care provider and the client can examine difficult issues and work toward a mutually beneficial solution. Barriers to care are varied and, along with moral and ethical issues, must be addressed to appropriately deliver spiritual care.

KEY CONCEPTS

1. A spiritual relationship between health care providers and clients can result in a sense of strength, inner peace, healing, harmonious interconnectedness, and meaning experienced by both parties.
2. Spiritual care can be provided by many different resources. Nurses, physicians, and social workers are spiritual care generalists, while chaplains, clergy, parish nurses, spiritual mentors, family and friends, and folk healers are considered spiritual care specialists.
3. While many health care providers may describe themselves as religious or spiritual, they may be inadequately prepared to administer effective spiritual care. One way for providers to effectively begin their spiritual education is to conduct a personal inventory of their own spirituality.
4. Barriers to providing spiritual care can include lack of education in spiritual care, lack of time, the presence of distractions, fear of invading a client's privacy, fear that spiritual care requires a mastery of the beliefs of each religious tradition, concerns about proselytizing to clients, and a lack of personal spiritual awareness.
5. Both spirituality and religion have shaped the moral and ethical framework of health care.

QUESTIONS FOR REFLECTION

1. Refer to the "The Spirituality of Health Care Providers" section of this chapter (pp. 32-33) and conduct a personal inventory of your own spirituality. What did you discover?

2. Suppose your patient/client has refused medical treatment for a life-threatening condition. With treatment, the client will recover; without it, the client will most likely die. How would you react and respond?

REFERENCES

Anandarajah, G., & Hight, E. (2001). Spirituality and medical practice: Using the HOPE questions as a practical tool for spiritual assessment. *American Family Physician, 63*(1), 81-89.

Association of Professional Chaplains. (2002). Board certified chaplain and requirements. Retrieved February 8, 2003, from http://www.professionalchaplains.org.

Bergquist, S., & King, J. (1994). Parish nursing: A conceptual framework. *Journal of Holistic Nursing, 12*(2), 155-170.

Boland, C. S. (1998). Parish nursing: Addressing the significance of social support and spirituality for sustained health-promoting behaviors in the elderly. *Journal of Holistic Nursing, 16*(3), 355-368.

Bonder, B., Martin, L., & Miracle, A. (2002). *Culture in clinical care.* Thorofare, NJ: SLACK Incorporated.

Boudreaux, E. D., O'Hea, E., & Chasuk, R. (2002). Spiritual role in healing: An alternative way of thinking. *Primary Care: Clinics in Office Practice, 29*(2), viii, 439-454.

Brush, B. L., & Daly, P. R. (2000). Assessing spirituality in primary care practice: Is there time? *Clinical Excellence for Nurse Practitioners, 4*(2), 67-71.

Burkhardt, M. A., & Nagai-Jacobson, M. G. (2002). *Spirituality: Living our connectedness.* Albany, NY: Delmar Thomson Learning.

Burkhardt, M. A., & Nathaniel, A. K. (1998). *Ethics and issues.* New York: Delmar Thomson Learning.

Carroll, G. A. (2002). Traditional medical cures along the Yukon. *Alaska Medicine, 44*(3), 66-69.

Cohen, K. (1998). Native American medicine. *Alternative Therapies, 4*(6), 45-57.

Davidhizar, R., Bechtel, G. A., & Juratovac, A. L. (2000). Responding to the cultural and spiritual needs of clients. *Journal of Practical Nursing, 50*(4), 20-23.

DeLashmutt, M., & Silva, M. C. (1998). The ethics of long-distance intercessory prayer. *Nursing Connections, 11*(4), 37-40.

Dossey, B. M. (2000). *Florence Nightingale: Mystic, visionary, healer.* Springhouse, PA: Springhouse.

Dossey, B. M., Keegan, L., & Guzzetta, C. E. (2000). *Holistic nursing: A handbook for practice* (3rd ed.). Gaithersburg, MD: Aspen.

Ebersole, P. (2000). Parish nurse leaders. *Geriatric Nursing, 21*(3), 148-149.

Engebretson, J. (1996). Comparison of nurses and alternative healers. *Image: Journal of Nursing Scholarship, 28*(2), 95-99.

Hatch, R. L., Burg, M. A., Naberhaus, D. S., & Hellmich, L. K. (1998). The Spiritual Involvement and Beliefs scale: Development and testing of a new instrument. *Journal of Family Practice, 46*(6), 476-486.

Hiatt, J. F. (1986). Spirituality, medicine, and healing. *Southern Medical Journal, 79*(6), 726-742.

Hitchcock, J. E., Schubert, P. E., & Thomas, S. A. (1999). *Community health nursing: Caring in action.* Albany: Delmar Thomson Learning.

Hodge, D. R. (2001). Spiritual assessment: A review of major qualitative methods and a new framework for assessing spirituality. *Social Work, 46*(3), 203-214.

Huch, M. H. (1999). Folk healers and nurse theorists. *Nursing Science Quarterly, 12*(3), 256.

Hurley, J. E. (1999). Breaking the spiritual care barrier. *Journal of Christian Nursing, 16*(3), 8-13.

Kleindienst, M. J. (1998). Spirituality: Where there is hope, there is life. *American Nephrology Nurses' Association Journal, 25*(4), 442.

Koenig, H. G. (2000). Spiritual aspects of surgery. *Ophthalmology Clinics of North America, 13*(1), 71-83.

Koenig, H. G. (2001). Religion, spirituality, and medicine: How are they related and what does it mean? *Mayo Clinic Proceedings, 76*(12), 1189-1191.

Kuebler, K. K., Berry, P. H., & Heidrich, D. E. (Eds.). (2002). *End of life care: Clinical practice guidelines.* New York: W. B. Saunders.

Larimore, W. L. (2001). Providing basic spiritual care for patients: Should it be the exclusive domain of pastoral professionals? *American Family Physician, 63*(1), 36, 38-40.

Larson, D. B., & Koenig, H. G. (2000). Is God good for your health? The role of spirituality in medical care. *Cleveland Clinic Journal of Medicine, 67*(2), 80-84.

Leetun, M. C. (1996). Wellness spirituality in the older adult: Assessment and intervention protocol. *Nurse Practitioner, 21*(8), 60, 65-70.

Lo, B. (2000). *Resolving ethical dilemmas: A guide for clinicians* (2nd ed.). Philadelphia: Lippincott, Williams & Wilkins.

Louis, M., & Alpert, P. (2000). Spirituality for nurses and their practice. *Nursing Leadership Forum, 5*(2), 43-49.

Macrae, J. (1995). Nightingale's spiritual philosophy and its significance for modern nursing. *Image: Journal of Nursing Scholarship, 27*(1), 8-10.

Mansen, T. J. (1993). The spiritual dimension of individuals: Conceptual development. *Nursing Diagnosis, 4*(4), 140-147.

Martsolf, D., & Mickley, J. (1998). The concept of spirituality in nursing theories: Differing worldviews and extent of focus. *Journal of Advanced Nursing, 27*(2), 294-303.

McSherry, W., & Cash, K. (2000). *Making sense of spirituality in nursing: An interactive approach.* Edinburgh: Churchill Livingstone.

McSherry, W., & Draper, P. (1998). The debates emerging from the literature surrounding the concept of spirituality as applied to nursing. *Journal of Advanced Nursing, 27*(4), 683-691.

McSherry, W., & Ross, L. (2002). Dilemmas of spiritual assessment: Considerations for nursing practice. *Journal of Advanced Nursing, 38*(5), 479-488.

Messikomer, C., & De Craemer, W. (2002). The spirituality of academic physicians: An ethnography of a scripture-based group in an academic medical center. *Academic Medicine, 77*(6), 562-573.

Miller, W. R. (Ed.). (1999). *Integrating spirituality into treatment.* Washington, DC: American Psychological Association.

Milne, D., & Howard, W. (2000). Rethinking the role of diagnosis in Navajo religious healing. *Medical Anthropology Quarterly, 14*(4), 543-570.

Mueller, P. S., Plevak, D. J., & Rummans, T. A. (2001). Religious involvement, spirituality, and medicine: Implications for clinical practice. *Mayo Clinic Proceedings, 76*(12), 1225-1235.

O'Brien, M. E. (1999). *Spirituality in nursing: Standing on holy ground.* Boston: Jones & Bartlett.

O'Connor, C. I. (2001). Characteristics of spirituality, assessment, and prayer in holistic nursing. *Nursing Clinics of North America, 36*(1), 33-42.

O'Hara, D. P. (2002). Is there a role for prayer and spirituality in health care? *Medical Clinics of North America, 86*(1), vi, 33-46.

Purtillo, R. (1999). *Ethical dimensions in the health professions.* Philadelphia: W. B. Saunders.

Rhi, B. Y. (2001). Culture, spirituality, and mental health: The forgotten aspects of religion and health. *Psychiatric Clinics of North America, 24*(3), ix-x, 569-579.

Salladay, S. A., & McDonnell, M. M. (1989). Spiritual care, ethical choices, and patient advocacy. *Nursing Clinics of North America, 24*(2), 543-549.

Shealey, C. N. (1999). *Sacred healing: The curing power of energy and spirituality.* Boston: Element Books.

Taylor, E. J. (2002). *Spiritual care: Nursing theory, research, and practice.* Upper Saddle River, NJ: Prentice Hall.

Thomas, C. L. (Ed.). (1997). *Taber's cyclopedic medical dictionary*. Philadelphia: F. A. Davis.

Thomason, C. L., & Brody, H. (1990). Inclusive spirituality. *Journal of Family Practice, 48*(2), 96-97.

Treloar, L. L. (2001). Is spiritual care ethical? *Journal of Christian Nursing, 18*(2), 16-20.

Trotter, R. T. (2001). Curanderismo: A picture of Mexican-American folk healing. *Journal of Alternative and Complementary Medicine, 7*(2), 129-131.

Tuck, I., Wallace, D., & Pullen, L. (2001). Spirituality and spiritual care provided by parish nurses. *Western Journal of Nursing Research, 23*(5), 441-453.

VandeCreek, L., & Burton, L. (2001). *Professional chaplaincy: Its role and importance in healthcare.* New York: Association for Clinical Pastoral Education, Association of Professional Chaplains, Canadian Association for Pastoral Practice and Education, National Association of Catholic Chaplains, National Association of Jewish Chaplains.

Walton, J. (1996). Spiritual relationships: A concept analysis. *Journal of Holistic Nursing, 14*(3), 237-250.

Wing, D. M. (1999). The aesthetics of caring: Where folk healers and nurse theorists converge. *Nursing Science Quarterly, 12*(3), 256-262.

Wright, K. B. (1998). Professional, ethical, and legal implications for spiritual care in nursing. *Image: Journal of Nursing Scholarship, 30*(1), 81-83.

Wright, M. C. (2002). The essence of spiritual care: A phenomenological enquiry. *Palliative Medicine, 16*(2), 125-132.

Zapata, J., & Shippee-Rice, R. (1999). The use of folk healing and healers by six Latinos living in New England: A preliminary study. *Journal of Transcultural Nursing, 19*(2), 136-142.

3

SPIRITUAL RITUALS

"Rituals... remind us that we all spring from the winter, the source,
the All-That-Is; that the aliveness of the Great Spirit lives in each of us;
and that we all have an equal place in things."
—Brook Medicine Eagle, in *Womanspirit*

LEARNING OBJECTIVES

Upon completing this chapter, you will be able to do the following:
1. Describe three phases of creating rituals.
2. Examine the spiritual ritual of prayer in health and healing.
3. Describe types and techniques of meditation, visualization, and guided imagery and describe their relationship to healing.
4. Explain the spiritual rituals of gratitude, spending time in nature, and art.
5. Describe the importance of storytelling in spiritual care.
6. Provide examples of why rituals work as a healing force.

INTRODUCTION

Through immigration, international travel, and globalization, spiritual journeys can take people down paths that were not available to previous generations. Today, people are exposed to many different religious practices, spiritual practices, and rituals that they may never have seen before. These practices often have specific meaning.

How does a spiritual practice differ from a ritual? While there is no one correct answer to the question, "What is a spiritual practice?," Scott (2001) provides the following perspective, demonstrating that most people view spiritual acts as part of everyday life:

- 91% of people see praying as a spiritual practice.
- 81% view attending worship services as a spiritual practice.
- 80% believe that parenting is a spiritual practice.
- 67% consider a walk in the forest to be a divine spiritual practice.
- 52% of adults affirm that making love is a spiritual practice.

Rituals, on the other hand, are practices that are often repeated and can provide a way for people to make life experiences meaningful. For example, rituals such as prayer and meditation may help individuals reconnect with their spirituality and thus support their spiritual health (Taylor, 2002). According to Dossey (1997), a ritual is an enactment of cultural beliefs and values:

- Rituals involve repetition and patterns of form and behaviors that have personal, healing value.
- Rituals are significant aspects of many religious traditions and cultures.
- They are spiritual acts.
- They can be any activities done with awareness.
- Rituals allow people to honor and celebrate life.
- They are sacred spaces of mind that honor the core of human experience and the power of the Invisible Force.
- They are rites of separation.
- They are a rich resource in caring for the spirit.
- Rituals contain steps for recovery and reducing anxiety, fear, and feelings of helplessness.

Rituals help awaken the spiritual self and help individuals connect with their inner core, other people, nature, and everything in the world. They help people to remember, to honor, and to change, and they can involve actions, symbols, and ceremonies. Rituals are a part of historical, religious, spiritual, and cultural traditions. *Traditional rituals* are handed down from one generation to another, while *self-generated rituals* are begun by an individual or group and have no cultural history or tradition. The basic elements of rituals include actions, meaningful patterns, intention, awareness, and purpose.

Rituals can be sacred or secular. Examples of sacred rituals might include saying grace at mealtime, religious worship, spiritual ceremony within any tradition, prayer, and meditation. Examples of secular rituals might include parades, family picnics, kissing under the mistletoe, or taking a daily walk for the purpose of exercise (Burkhardt & Nagai-Jacobson, 2002).

The following sections will look at how rituals are created, then at the specific types of rituals and why they work as a healing force.

CREATING RITUALS

There are many types of rituals, but an important aspect of healing is creating personalized rituals. According to Achterberg, Dossey, and Kolkmeier (1994), creating personalized rituals incorporates three phases:

1. **The separation phase:** Begins when the individual starts to relax, creates a positive healing intention for the experience, and then enters a healing state of consciousness.

2. **The transition phase:** Occurs when the individual becomes attuned to the relaxation process; uses imagery or imagination; and integrates the senses of sight, hearing, taste, touch, and smell with the condition that needs healing.
3. **The return phase:** Occurs when the individual gently returns to a wakeful state, experiences a deeper sense of relaxation, and feels renewed energy.

When preparing for a ritual, the individual (or health care provider) can support its healing aspects by doing the following (Achterberg et al., 1994):

- Taking care of basic comfort needs.
- Making sure the environment is supportive to the process (e.g., comfortable temperature, subtle lighting, soothing colors, etc.).
- Creating a sacred space or room.
- Having all necessary materials available (e.g., candles, incense, music, etc.).
- Making sure there are no distractions or interruptions.

The key to providing spiritual care is communicating with clients to determine if they are comfortable using specific rituals and then working with them to design or incorporate a ritual that is healing for them.

PRAYER

People throughout the ages perceived a relationship between spiritual practices and health and healing long before modern science began. Although the power of prayer in health and healing cannot be underestimated, it has only recently been acknowledged by modern science (Dossey, 1993, 1999, 2001; Koenig, 1999; Matthews & Clark, 1998). Today, health care professionals are beginning to look beyond traditional ethics and science to better understand the power of prayer and the health effects of spirituality (Silva & DeLashmutt, 1998). Research has demonstrated that regular prayer, scripture reading, or study has provided health benefits (Koenig, 1999; Matthews, 2000). Research on the biological effects of prayer and spiritual healing is constantly growing and includes studies on micro-organisms, plants, cancer cells, animals, and humans (Brown-Saltzman, 1997; Dossey, 1993; Matthews, 2000).

What Is Prayer?

Prayer has meaning for many individuals. It is the most common form of spiritual ritual and is practiced by religious as well as nonreligious individuals throughout the world. Virtually every culture prays in one form or another, especially during times of stress and at the end of life (O'Hara, 2002). Even in Buddhism, which does not believe in a "person God" as creator, prayers are a central component.

An expression of the spirit, prayer both influences and is affected by an individual's spirituality (Meraviglia, 1999). It represents a desire to communicate with God or a Higher Power. Dossey, Keegan, and Guzzetta (2000) define prayer as "a deep human instinct that flows from the core of one's being where the longing for and awareness of one's connectedness with the source of life are blended" (p. 99). Dossey (2001) offers this broad and inclusive definition of prayer: "Prayer is communication with the Absolute" (p. 224).

With a wide variety of forms and expressions, prayer is part of many religious traditions and rituals. It may be individual or communal and public or private.

Sometimes prayer is a conscious activity and at other times it is less conscious. Elements of prayer include speaking (often silently), listening, waiting, and being silent. Prayer also includes adoration, confession, invocation, intercession, lamentation, and thanksgiving (Dossey, 1993, 2001; Dossey et al., 2000).

Dossey (1993) confirms that prayer is remarkably democratic, that no particular religion holds a monopoly on prayer's efficacy, and that one does not need to be religious to pray effectively or to benefit medically from prayer. Although the exact mechanism is unknown, evidence supports that prayer works (Dossey, 1993, 2001; Taylor, 2002). Dossey (1993) proposes that prayer is "nonlocal" (i.e., not confined by time or space) and is derived from quantum physics.

Techniques for Praying

Many techniques are used in praying, including the following (Capps, 1993; Dossey, 1993; Fontaine, 2000; O'Conner, 2001; Taylor, 2002):

- Relaxation, quieting, and breath awareness
- Attention training and focusing
- Imagery and visualization
- Intentionality
- Movement, such as dancing, walking, or drumming
- Inspirational or sacred readings
- Anointing with oil
- Singing
- Meditation
- Music
- Chanting

Types of Prayer

There are many ways of developing a daily spiritual practice of prayer and many effective ways to pray for one's self and others. Types of prayer may include petitionary, intercessory, adoration, ritual, meditative or contemplative, and colloquial (Dossey, 2001; Dossey et al., 2000; Holt-Ashley, 2000; Levin, 1996; Macrae, 2001; Matthews & Clark, 1998; Taylor, 2002).

- **Petitionary prayer:** Involves asking a Higher Power to respond to a specific request, usually for personal healing.
- **Intercessory prayer:** Often called "distant prayer," it is petitionary prayer on behalf of others, with or without their knowledge. It occurs when one person prays for someone else to receive something. Usually this involves praying for someone else's health.
- **Adoration prayer:** Involves praising and glorifying a Higher Power. This type of prayer is an affirmation of the loving energy within and without one's self. It transcends the ego and involves turning one's life over to a Higher Power. This is not an avoidance of responsibility but rather a positive surrender to a Higher Power and a willingness to do what has to be done for healing to take place.

- **Ritual prayer:** Involves using spiritual readings, repetition, or formal prayers or rites, like a rosary or a prayer book. Ritual prayer involves the repetition of prayers created by another and is often found in religious literature.
- **Meditative prayer or contemplative prayer:** Involves listening for the "still small voice within" and having a sense of openness toward the divine independence of thoughts and words. The purpose is to objectively observe one's self becoming absorbed in the unity of being, to experience one's unity with a Higher Power, and to experience life as it unfolds. Meditative or contemplative prayer involves the opening of the mind and heart to a Higher Power that transcends words or thoughts. This type of prayer exists in all the great religious traditions of the world.
- **Colloquial prayer:** Involves communicating with the divine in an informal, honest, and self-revealing manner as if talking to a friend. This type of prayer is used to seek directions and guidance in making a decision.

Prayer and Healing

Prayer can profoundly affect the healing process. Research demonstrates that religious practices such as worship attendance and prayer may contribute to physical and emotional health. Although the studies have not demonstrated a cause-and-effect relationship, there is strong evidence of an important connection between religious practice and good health (Fontaine, 2000; Taylor, 2002). As Taylor (2002) writes, "Although experimental evidence of prayer's curative effect is inconclusive, there have been several correlational studies that demonstrate relationships between prayer and psychological health benefits" (p. 207).

In addition to turning to medical care for their healing, people also turn to prayer. According to Matthews & Clark (1998):

- **People cope with illness** through a learned process by using prayer and other forms of spiritual involvement when they are not completely cured of their illness.
- **Individuals may experience the arrest of the progression of illnesses** with diseases such as cancer and heart disease.
- **Individuals may experience remission or complete healing of illnesses** through the combination of prayer and medical care.

Matthews and Clark (1998) explain the impact of prayer in this way:

Of course, we know that the faith factor is not a panacea—the mortality rate for human beings still remains 100%. But even when physical healing does not occur, some degree of improvement almost always takes place, most often a sense of peace in facing a serious illness or disability. (p. 61)

Prayer and the Health Care Provider

Health care providers can incorporate prayer into the care of their clients. Health care professionals who are aware of individual ways of praying and meditating can help the patient or client consider the meaning of prayer in his or her life and explore ways to reach out to his or her God or Higher Power during times of health care crises.

Praying with clients is an intimate act and should be approached carefully and respectfully. It is important to pray in an appropriate manner. For example, a brief assessment of the client's prayer habits and beliefs is necessary prior to praying with that client. Other suggestions for praying with clients include the following (Holt-Ashley, 2000; Taylor, 2002):

- Obtain permission from the client prior to praying with him or her.
- Create personalized conversational prayers that reflect the client's current concern.
- Match the type of prayer experience with the client's personality, preference, and current circumstance.
- Establish privacy by closing doors or curtains.
- Observe the client's response.

Prayer as a ritual can be healing and comforting. However, the health care provider should understand that praying may not be appropriate for everyone. If a client refuses prayer, the health care provider should not attempt to force personal beliefs on the client.

MEDITATION, VISUALIZATION, AND GUIDED IMAGERY

*"Meditation is simply about being yourself and knowing about who that is.
It is about coming to realize that you are on a path whether you like it or not,
namely the path that is your life."*
—Jon Kabat-Zinn

Meditation originated in ancient India about 3,000 years ago and has existed in some form in most major religions and many secular organizations. It is often distinguished from prayer by the lack of directedness toward the divine (Barrows & Jacobs, 2002). Because many individuals regularly practice meditation in a prescribed manner, it can also be considered a ritual and a process to spiritual transformation (Taylor, 2002).

Meditation is a learned skill. When practiced in a disciplined manner, it provides many physiological benefits, such as stress reduction, decreased adrenaline flow, lowered metabolic rate, decreased heart rate, improved immune and cardiovascular function, relaxation, and decreased pain. The regular practice of meditation may lead to new insights about life issues, heightened creativity, inspiration, greater compassion for others, and a greater connection to one's own inner guidance (Achterberg et al., 1994; Reynolds, 2001).

There are many ways to meditate and many different forms of meditation, but they all share the characteristic of intentionally training a person's attention and concentration. All meditative techniques involve conscious breathing and a focus on what is happening in each present moment until the mind becomes empty of thoughts, judgments, and past and future concerns (Dossey et al., 2000; Reynolds, 2001).

Meditation can be performed while sitting, lying down, walking, or jogging. Examples of meditation practices include mindfulness meditation, transcendental meditation (TM), and relaxation response meditation. Another type of meditation is moving meditation. Yoga, Qi Gong, therapeutic touch, Sufi dancing, and Native American and shamanic ritual dance are all examples of moving mediation practices.

Meditation can be an intensely spiritual experience. To enter into a meditative state, the following three methods may be helpful: breathing techniques, meditating with sound, and meditating with visualization (Reynolds, 2001).

Breathing Techniques

Using breathing techniques is one of the simplest meditation practices and an important component of most forms of meditation. Breathing techniques involve counting each breath while breathing in and out. Each inhalation and exhalation together count as one breath. Usually, the individual breathes in slowly through the nose (counting from the number 1 to 10) and breathes out slowly through the mouth (counting backward from the number 10 to 1).

Another method is a technique called spaced breathing. This involves taking as much time as possible between breaths. The individual breathes gently and slowly and counts to 5 for each inhalation, holds the breath for a count of 5, and then exhales to a count of 5 (Dossey et al., 2000; Reynolds, 2001; Taylor, 2002).

Meditating With Sound

Other forms of meditation use mantras, chanting, singing bowls, drums, and audiotapes to incorporate sound vibrations in the promotion of a meditative state of mind (Dossey et al., 2000; Reynolds, 2001).

- **Mantras** involve synchronizing the breathing with the silent repetition of a sound, word, or phrase (such as sacred Sanskrit syllables and words such as "om").
- **Chanting** involves repeating certain words or sounds aloud
- **Singing bowls** (usually made of a unique alloy or quartz crystal) are rubbed or struck with a wooden stick to create soothing sounds that invoke a meditative state.
- **Drums** are beaten in rhythm with the breath or heartbeat to create a deep meditative state.
- **Audiotapes** of music, nature sounds, or meditation instructions can help create a relaxed meditative state.

Meditating With Visualization

The use of visualization techniques—another form of meditation—can include picturing a sacred place, focusing on an external object, or visualizing sacred symbols (Reynolds, 2001; Taylor, 2002).

- **Picturing a sacred place** may involve picturing a real or imaginary place, such as a stream with water flowing over the boulders, a mountain landscape, an ocean scene, or the image of a forest. Contemplating this scene "transports" the individual to a meditative state.
- **Focusing on an external object** may involve keeping the eyes open and focusing on a single object (such as a candle flame) for a specific period of time.
- **Visualizing sacred symbols** involves visualizing certain symbols and shapes regarded as sacred by many cultures. For example, Hindus and Buddhists use a mandala, a graphic representation depicting the universe. Sacred symbols can help individuals connect with their deep subconscious awareness and create a meditative state.

A Simple Meditation

Sit comfortably erect with your eyes closed while paying attention to your breathing. Observe yourself inhaling and exhaling, allowing whatever thoughts you may have to leave your mind. In the beginning, your mind may wander, so each time this occurs, gently refocus on your breathing. To prevent your mind from wandering, try silently repeating a word, or mantra, such as love or peace. You will eventually experience longer periods of silence between each thought.

This technique should be practiced 10 to 20 minutes, once or twice a day. With commitment and practice, the benefits of mediation will become apparent (Dossey et al., 2000; Reynolds, 2001; Taylor, 2002).

Guided Imagery

Barrows and Jacobs (2002) describe guided imagery as "the imaginative capacity of the mind to affect one's physical, emotional, and spiritual state" (p. 18). Imagery has been defined as the thought process that invokes and uses the senses of vision, hearing, smell, taste, movement, position, and touch. It is the communication mechanism between perception, emotion, and bodily change (Achterberg et al., 1994; Brown-Saltzman, 1997). By using guided imagery, individuals can develop new patterns or ways of seeing, facilitate problem solving, and create a sense of control over their inner and outer life.

Closely related to hypnosis, guided imagery has a presuggestion phase, which includes relaxation and the focus of attention; a suggestion phase, which usually involves images; and a postsuggestion reinforcement phase. The underlying premise is that an individual's physiology and psychology are altered during hypnosis. Guided imagery has been investigated in the following areas (Barrows & Jacobs, 2002):

- Quality of life with a chronic illness, such as cancer.
- Treatment of chronic pain.
- Improvement of surgery outcomes.

Guided imagery may have diverse applications in health care in the areas of infertility, childbirth, chronic and acute pain, psychotherapy, and grief work.

GRATITUDE

"Gratitude unlocks the fullness of life. It turns what we have into enough, and more.
It turns denial into acceptance, chaos to order, confusion to clarity.
It can turn a meal into a feast, a house into a home, a stranger into a friend.
Gratitude makes sense of our past, brings peace for today,
and creates a vision for tomorrow."
—Melody Beattie

The spiritual practice of gratitude is a powerful force and can be a state of mind as well as a way of life. Being grateful for what one has, instead of worrying about what one lacks, enables the individual to let go of negative thoughts and attitudes and reduce stress, anxiety, and depression. Burkhardt and Nagai-Jacobson (2002) describe the origin of gratitude this way, "Our experience of grace as a blessing that comes into our lives unearned, without merit, calls forth the response of gratitude" (p. 71).

One way to practice gratitude is to focus on the positive aspects of life. This can be accomplished by keeping a gratitude journal—an inventory of all the positive things that occur each day, week, and month. Keeping such a journal can set the stage for living a life that is more connected to spirit (Fontaine, 2000).

Engaging in an act of gratitude may often restore balance and perspective (Burkhardt & Nagai-Jacobson, 2002; Fontaine, 2000). Grateful acts might include any or all of the following:

- Making a list of things you are grateful for in your life.
- Creating opportunities to help others.
- Calling a special friend.
- Being aware that life is a gift.
- Saying grace before meals.
- Engaging in daily prayers.
- Always remembering to say thank you when someone helps you, gives you a compliment, or gives you a gift.

SPENDING TIME IN NATURE

Have you ever been moved by the site of a spectacular sunset? Have you ever walked barefoot through leaves and experienced their rustling and crunching sounds beneath your feet? Experiencing the pleasure of the natural environment—whether it be a deserted beach, a shimmering wheat field, a majestic mountain, a vivid sky at sunset, a lush forest, a beautiful waterfall, or a quiet stream—may be considered a spiritual experience. The desire for aesthetic pleasure on a deep level is a strong human craving, and aesthetic experiences, or even the act of contemplating nature, can confer numerous health benefits (Matthews & Clark, 1998; Taylor, 2002).

Throughout history, most religious, spiritual, and cultural traditions have had strong connections and relationships with nature. According to Taylor (2002), "Many religious traditions consider nature, or the outdoors and its world of living things, to be the handiwork or a literal illustration of God" (p. 262). For example, Native American religious traditions express a positive relationship to nature that is called nature-centered spirituality. It is found in many other religious traditions worldwide (Dossey, 1997).

Being in natural environments and viewing or experiencing nature can foster reconnection with the self physically, emotionally, and spiritually. Nature is the most visible manifestation of Spirit, whereby individuals interact with primal energies in the forms of earth, water, fire, and air (Ruffing, 1997; Taylor, 2002).

- **Earth:** To connect with nature and the earth, individuals can take a walk in a park, hike through the woods, garden, ride a bike, camp, or take a sailing trip. Spending time in nature helps to restore balance in one's life and, at the same time, deepens the connection with spirit.
- **Water:** Spending time near or in the water can contribute to feelings of well-being. Swimming in the ocean, a lake, or a river, as well as soaking in a mineral hot spring, are excellent ways to benefit from this life-enhancing energy.

- **Fire:** Exposure to fire around a campground or before a fireplace may have health benefits. To Native Americans, fire is an important part of the vision quest ritual used to connect with the Great Spirit.
- **Air:** Exposure to air is a potent force for restoring energy and for connecting with Spirit as it flows through the body. Of all of nature's elements, air may be the purest manifestation of Spirit. Air is essential to life and health on all levels.

Earth Elements

We live in air, but we do not see it, forgetting to show our thanks for the breath that gives us life.

Our bodies are made of the elements of earth, but few recognize the essential energy of the Earth Mother that fuels our physical strength.

Water blends our dreams and feelings into a sacred creative drive called the will, but few have learned to master free will or the flow of Creation.

Our hearts contain fire, the Eternal Flame of Love, but few have learned how to use its light to illuminate their paths.

These elements give us the ability to touch our primal human natures and the potential of our spirits, seeing both as being equally sacred. (Sams, 1994)

Helping clients experience a positive connection with nature promotes spiritual health as well as other dimensions of physical health. Approaches to using nature as a resource in providing spiritual care may include the following (Taylor, 2002):

- Providing a window view of natural surroundings.
- Displaying an aquarium of beautiful fish.
- Providing access to animals or an animal-assisted therapy program.
- Providing flower boxes in a client's room.
- Displaying photographs, pictures, or illustrations that depict natural settings.

ART

The origin of art lies in religion and spirituality. Used as a healing force, the arts have been around since the beginning of humankind, with the earliest humans using pictures, stories, dances, and chants as healing rituals. Art has been called an expression of the soul, and it is experiencing renewed interest as an important aspect of the spirit. The arts are now viewed as an integral component of holistic and spiritual care (Bailey, 1997; Rollins & Riccio, 2002).

Art can be a powerful tool in promoting healing even when a cure is no longer an option. For many, healing art is a spiritual path, a transformational process, and a way of being. Many individuals find that the numerous forms of art are doors to, and expressions of, the spirit (Dossey et al., 2000; Tate & Longo, 2002; Taylor, 2002).

Art can nurture the spirit and can take the following forms (Dossey et al., 2000; Rollins & Riccio, 2002; Tate & Longo, 2002; Taylor, 2002):

- Drawing
- Painting
- Sculpting

- Cooking
- Sewing
- Designing and building
- Conducting a symphony
- Listening to or creating music
- Writing or reading literature
- Writing or reading poetry
- Puppetry
- Dancing
- Drumming
- Gardening
- Storytelling

Engaging in these activities may provide a sense of accomplishment or the opportunity to be creative, which—in itself—expresses spirituality, connects people to other cultures, or provides a means of transcendence. Art aids in healing in various ways (Taylor, 2002):

- It releases inner images that increase self-awareness.
- It helps make sense of experiences.
- It provides the viewer of art objects with a means for accessing mental images of healing.

Artists can play an important role as part of the interdisciplinary team in providing spiritual care in the health care setting. A specialized form of therapy called art therapy is discussed in Chapter 7.

STORYTELLING

Within the United States, there is a resurgent interest in the use of storytelling for both clinical practice and research (Banks-Wallace, 1999). According to Lawlis (1995), storytelling is an "art developed during the beginnings of human history, probably to teach the wisdom of generations past, including basic mental and physical health principles" (p. 40). The art of storytelling is a human phenomenon. It is an intrinsic component of most cultures, and it is a means of preserving common characteristics of a culture and passing them to subsequent generations (Anderson, 1998; Banks-Wallace, 1999; Rice, 1999).

History, values, and cultures are often preserved through storytelling. In addition, storytelling promotes critical thinking, enhances communication, improves education, inspires creativity, strengthens collegiality and collaboration, builds self-esteem and rapport, enhances human sensitivity skills, and helps a person to understand and explain his or her unique view of the meaning of life (Anderson, 1998; Bowles, 1995; Kirkpatrick, Ford, & Castelloe, 1997; Lindesmith & McWeeny, 1994).

A story has been defined as a narrative of events arranged in a time sequence, as a way of knowing. A story unifies singular, disconnected elements of life experience into a whole, and it provides a descriptive account of human experience as told by its original storyteller (Anderson, 1998; Taylor, 1997). A story is about characters, relationships, plots, places, and events. In the health care setting, stories are embedded in everyday conversations (Anderson, 1998). Sharing stories with clients and colleagues is a natural way of connecting and communicating caring (Rice, 1999).

Storytelling is both an art and a science. However, according to Lawlis (1995), a story has four basic features that are essential to its success:

1. The way the storyteller tells the story.
2. The relaxation skills achieved by concentrating on the story.
3. The imagery of an obstacle or challenge to the hero.
4. The participation of the listener.

Storytelling nurtures the spirit and can include life reviews, reminiscence, and oral stories. The health care provider who plans to use storytelling needs to make it a meaningful experience for participants. Because storytelling promotes spiritual as well as physical well-being, these guidelines for storytelling may be helpful (Lindesmith & McWeeny, 1994; Taylor, 1997):

- Create an environment that is conducive to storytelling by providing a comfortable area for the participants.
- Plan group size according to the amount of time allowed for the story so participants can share and reflect on the story and its message.
- Darken the room slightly and avoid interruptions while the story and discussions are in progress.
- Provide oral or written directions to participants.
- Invite participants to voluntarily share stories.
- Help participants to connect the story to the present context.
- Ask participants to use their best listening skills and attentiveness.
- Initiate a group discussion about the experience so participants can gain a deeper understanding of the story.

Analyzing the Story

When all stories have been shared in a group, the following questions can help the facilitator initiate a group discussion about the process of storytelling, not about the stories that were told. The following questions may help in describing the experience (Lindesmith & McWeeny, 1994; Taylor, 1997):

- What values and beliefs are revealed in the story?
- What was your storytelling experience?
- What are the applications for storytelling in your life?
- What life themes emerged in the story?
- Why did the story get told now?

Storytelling, a valuable tool, can help health care providers be truly client-focused and help in planning and providing spiritual care. Health care providers can incorporate storytelling into practice by being aware of the following (Burkhardt & Nagai-Jacobson, 2002, p. 311):

- Recognize that each person (including the health care provider) is an ongoing, unfinished story.
- Understand your own stories and their influence on the hearing of another person's story.
- Appreciate the breadth and depth of another person's story, even though you can know only a brief part of the story that has brought another to this particular time and place.
- Recognize connections and relationships that enhance the understanding of the story.

- Develop an understanding of the theory and research on the story as related to health care.
- Elicit and listen for and to the stories of others.

RITUALS AS A HEALING FORCE

Achterberg et al. (1994) writes, "Healing rituals both reflect and create the values of an individual and a culture" (p. 4). During the experience of an illness, which challenges the whole being—physical, emotional, mental, and spiritual—rituals help individuals to connect with the deeper resources within themselves and with family, community, Divine Spirit, strength, and wisdom. This connection supports and contributes to the healing process (Burkhardt & Nagai-Jacobson, 2002).

Healing rituals have been developed over decades or centuries and, based on trial and error, are deemed to be successful. Achterberg et al. (1994, pp. 13-19) provide examples of why rituals may work as a healing force:

- Rituals contain steps for recovery through highly structured practices, which include rules and prescriptions for behavior.
- They reduce anxiety and depression by substituting meaningful and creative activity for nonconstructive worrying.
- They reduce feelings of helplessness through repetitive actions that clear and quiet the mind and allow for closer spiritual connections.
- They allow for demonstration of family and community support through presence, love, and bonding during the time of crisis; through loving attention and care by the self and others; and by offering an opportunity to renew and reframe beliefs and concepts about the self.
- They encourage self-acceptance and compassion by helping individuals feel special or worthy and believe and trust in themselves.
- They may directly evoke a Higher Power or healing source through divine intervention, intercessory prayer, the healing power of love, and energy forces for healing.

Health care professionals can support the power of rituals by providing opportunities for their clients to consider and experience the use of rituals in their lives. Regardless of the form they take, rituals provide a way for individuals to find meaning in their life experiences. Rituals also provide spiritual support, thus enabling people to change, heal, believe, and celebrate (Dossey et al., 2000; Taylor, 2002).

SUMMARY

The spiritual rituals of prayer, meditation, guided imagery, gratitude, spending time in nature, and art help people connect to their inner being, to others, and to the Divine Spirit. A part of spiritual and cultural traditions, rituals help to provide awareness, meaning, intention, and purpose in life. Health care professionals and spiritual care providers can incorporate the use of spiritually-healing rituals in the care of their clients and for themselves.

KEY CONCEPTS

1. Rituals help people connect with their inner core, other people, nature, and everything in the world and help them to remember, honor, and change. They can involve actions, symbols, and ceremonies.
2. Prayer is the most common form of spiritual ritual practiced by religious as well as nonreligious individuals throughout the world. The power of prayer and healing has now been acknowledged by modern science.
3. Meditation and guided imagery have diverse applications in health care and can provide physiological, psychological, and spiritual benefits.
4. The spiritual practice of gratitude may restore balance and perspective and alleviate stress, anxiety, and depression in an individual's life.
5. Spending time in nature nurtures the spirit and contributes to positive health outcomes.
6. Art as a healing force is an important aspect of the spirit and is an expression of the soul.
7. Storytelling nurtures the spirit, promotes critical thinking, enhances communication, and helps an individual to understand and explain meaning in life.

QUESTIONS FOR REFLECTION

1. Take a few minutes to think about the rituals or spiritual practices you use in your own life. In what ways do they help you connect with your spirituality or support your spiritual health?
2. Everyone has unique gifts and abilities that can be utilized in developing spiritual practices and rituals. Some people are natural storytellers, while others have artistic or musical ability. What gifts, talents, or abilities could you utilize to help your clients with their spiritual practices or healing rituals?

REFERENCES

Achterberg, J., Dossey, B., & Kolkmeier, L. (1994). *Rituals of healing: Using imagery for health and wellness*. New York: Bantam Books.

Anderson, G. (1998). Storytelling: A holistic foundation for genetic nursing. *Holistic Nursing Practice, 12*(3), 64-74.

Bailey, S. S. (1997). The arts in spiritual care. *Seminars in Oncology Nursing, 13*(4), 242-247.

Banks-Wallace, J. (1999). Storytelling as a tool for providing holistic care to women. *American Journal of Maternal Child Nursing, 24*(1), 20-24.

Barrows, K. A., & Jacobs, B. P. (2002). Mind-body medicine: An introduction and review of the literature. *Medical Clinics of North America, 86*(1), 11-33.

Bowles, N. (1995). Story-telling: A search for meaning within nursing practice. *Nurse Education Today, 15*(5), 365-369.

Brown-Saltzman, K. (1997). Replenishing the spirit by meditative prayer and guided imagery. *Seminars in Oncology Nursing, 13*(4), 255-259.

Burkhardt, M. A., & Nagai-Jacobson, M. G. (2002). *Spirituality: Living our connectedness*. New York: Delmar Thomson Learning.

Capps, D. (1993). Praying in our own behalf: Toward the revitalization of petitionary prayer. *Second Opinion, 19*(1), 21-39.

Dossey, B. M. (1997). *Core curriculum for holistic nursing*. Gaithersburg, MD: Aspen.

Dossey, B. M., Keegan, L., & Guzzetta, C. E. (2000). *Holistic nursing: A handbook for practice* (3rd ed.). Gaithersburg, MD: Aspen.

Dossey, L. (1993). *Healing words: The power of prayer and the practice of medicine*. San Francisco: HarperCollins.

Dossey, L. (1999). Do religion and spirituality matter in health? A response to the recent article in *The Lancet*. *Alternative Therapies, 5*(3), 16-18.

Dossey, L. (2001). *Healing beyond the body: Medicine and the infinite reach of the mind*. Boston: Shambhala.

Fontaine, K. L. (2000). *Healing practices: Alternative therapies for nursing*. Upper Saddle River, NJ: Prentice Hall.

Holt-Ashley, M. (2000). Nurses pray: Use of prayer and spirituality as a complementary therapy in the intensive care setting. *AACN Clinical Issues: Advance Practice in Acute Critical Care, 11*(1), 60-67.

Kirkpatrick, M. K., Ford, S., & Castelloe, B. P. (1997). Storytelling: An approach to client-centered care. *Nurse Educator, 22*(2), 38-40.

Koenig, H. G. (1999). *The healing power of faith: Science explores medicine's last great frontier*. New York: Simon & Schuster.

Lawlis, G. F. (1995). Storytelling as therapy: Implications for medicine. *Alternative Therapies, 1*(2), 40-45.

Levin, J. S. (1996). How prayer heals: A theoretical model. *Alternative Therapies, 2*(1), 66-73.

Lindesmith, K. A., & McWeeny, M. (1994). The power of storytelling. *Journal of Continuing Education in Nursing, 25*(4), 186-187.

Macrae, J. A. (2001). *Nursing as a spiritual practice: A contemporary application of Florence Nightingale's views*. New York: Springer.

Matthews, D. A. (2000). Prayer and spirituality. *Rheumatic Diseases of North America, 26*(1), 177-187.

Matthews, D. A., & Clark, C. (1998). *The faith factor: Proof of the healing power of prayer*. New York: Penguin Books.

Meraviglia, M. G. (1999). Critical analysis of spirituality and its empirical indicators. *Journal of Holistic Nursing, 17*(1), 18-33.

O'Conner, C. I. (2001). Characteristics of spirituality, assessment, and prayer in holistic nursing. *Holistic Nursing Care, 36*(1), 33-45.

O'Hara, D. P. (2002). Is there a role for prayer and spirituality in health care? *Medical Clinics of North America, 86*(1), 33-46.

Reynolds, C. (2001). *Spiritual fitness*. London: Thorsons.

Rice, R. (1999). A little art in home care: Poetry and storytelling for the soul. *Geriatric Nursing, 20*(3), 165-166.

Rollins, J. A., & Riccio, L. L. (2002). ART is the heART: A palette of possibilities for hospice. *Pediatric Nursing, 28*(4), 355-362.

Ruffing, J. (1997). "To have been one with the earth...": Nature in contemporary Christian mystical experience. *Presence: The Journal of Spiritual Directors International, 3*(1), 40-54.

Sams, J. (1994). *Earth medicine: Ancestors' ways of harmony for many moons*. New York: HarperCollins.

Scott, R. O. (2001). A look in the mirror: Finding our way in this new spiritual landscape. *Spirituality and Aging, 4*(1), 26.

Silva, M. C., & DeLashmutt, M. (1998). Spirituality and prayer: A New Age paradigm for ethics. *Nursing Connections, 11*(2), 13-17.

Tate, F. B., & Longo, D. A. (2002). Art therapy: Enhancing psychosocial nursing. *Journal of Psychosocial Nursing, 40*(3), 40-47.

Taylor, E. J. (1997). The story behind the story: The use of storytelling in spiritual caregiving. *Seminars in Oncology Nursing, 13*(4), 252-254.

Taylor, E. J. (2002). *Spiritual care*. Upper Saddle River, NJ: Prentice Hall.

4

SPIRITUALITY, RELIGION, AND HEALTH

"Health is my expected heaven."
—John Keats

LEARNING OBJECTIVES

Upon completing this chapter, you will be able to do the following:
1. Describe the concepts of religion and religiosity.
2. Identify the connection between spirituality, religion, and health.
3. Describe major spiritual elements and rituals found in Buddhism, Hinduism, Islam, Judaism, and Christianity.
4. Discuss the benefits of religion on specific health care conditions.

INTRODUCTION

Spirituality and religion are similar in many aspects and have overlapping concepts. Experientially, they both involve transcendence, connectedness, and the search for meaning and purpose (Coyle, 2002; Mueller, Plevak, & Rummans, 2001). However, the two terms also have distinct differences.

Spirituality involves an integrative energy in that it "encompasses all aspects of human being and is a means of experiencing life" (Goddard, 2000, p. 975). To many, spirituality is experiential, not intellectual. It can be manifested in experiences with nature or animals, or in relationships with others, the self, or a divine being (Macrae, 2001).

Matthews & Clark (1998) propose the following distinctions between spirituality and religion:

- Religion focuses on establishing community, while spirituality focuses on individual growth.
- Religion is easier to identify and objectively measure than spirituality.
- Religion is more formal in worship, more authoritarian in its directions, more orthodox and systematic in doctrine, and has more formally prescribed and proscribed behaviors than spirituality.
- While religion is more behavior-based and focused on outward, observable practices, spirituality is more emotion-based and focused on inner experiences.
- While religion is particular, segregating one group from another, spirituality is more universal, emphasizing community and unity with others.

"In short, spirituality poses questions; religion composes answers" (Matthews & Clark, 1998, p. 182).

This chapter explores the connection between spirituality, religion, and health and examines some of the spiritual elements and rituals found in the world's major religions. Before proceeding further, however, it is important to define the terms *religion* and *religiosity*.

RELIGION AND RELIGIOSITY

Religion is usually recognized as the practical expression of spirituality; the organization, rituals, and practice of one's beliefs. Derived from the Latin word *religare*, which means to bind together (Mueller et al., 2001), religion is a personal way of expressing spirituality through affiliations, rites, and rituals based upon creeds and communal practices (Matthews & Clark, 1998). Religion is composed of beliefs and willful behaviors with a moral component. It can be intertwined with a culture, as Judaism is with Israel or Hinduism is with India, or it may be countercultural, as with the Amish in the United States (Burkhardt & Nathaniel, 1998). According to Boudreaux, O'Hea, and Chasuk (2002), religion "searches for the sacred and uses specific, prescribed behaviors and practices sanctioned by an identifiable group of people" (p. 440).

Religion and its accompanying beliefs and behaviors can affect every aspect of life, including social organizations, political beliefs, economic status, family life, sexual activity, criminal behavior, fertility, personality characteristics, human development, and even the report of paranormal experiences (Levin, Chatters, Ellison, & Taylor, 1996). People with an intrinsic religious orientation internalize their religious doctrines and follow them completely. Religion is a major force in their lives. People with an extrinsic religious orientation regard religion as a means to provide security or social connections in their lives (Mickley, Soeken, & Belcher, 1992).

Religiosity is a term that refers to the degree of participation in or adherence to the beliefs and practices of an organized religion (Mueller et al., 2001). Religiosity is a more public, human-made, formal, and socialized practice, while spirituality is a private, naturally occurring, informal practice that exists independently of any formal institutions (Boudreaux et al., 2002). Religiosity may be expressed through dietary practices, prayers, rituals, modes of dress, and the study of sacred texts (Dossey, 1993, 1996).

While an individual might be spiritual without being religious, or religious without being spiritual, the very spiritual tend to be religious, and the very religious tend to be spiritual. Many people, whether they are religious or not, are aware of an evolving pattern of life that is out of their control and links them in a personally meaningful way to the rest of reality. They also report feeling the presence of God (or a Higher Power) in nature, and this feeling connects them creatively to others (Narayanasamy, 1999).

American Spirituality and Religion

No amount of data can capture the full complexity of the terms *religious* and *spiritual*, but the following information may help to explain American spirituality and religion (Larson & Koenig, 2000; Matthews, 2000; Scott, 2001):

- 59% of Americans describe themselves as both religious and spiritual.
- 65% of Americans have positive associations with the word *religion*.
- 74% of Americans associate the word *spirituality* with positive feelings.
- 20% of Americans see themselves as solely spiritual.
- 8% of Americans see themselves as solely religious.
- Approximately 95% of Americans believe in God or a Higher Power.
- More than 40% of Americans attend worship services weekly.
- Approximately 75% of Americans state that their religious faith forms the foundation for their approach to life.
- 73% of Americans report that prayer is an important part of their daily life.
- 35% of Americans engage in prayer for the healing of their medical conditions.

THE CONNECTION BETWEEN SPIRITUALITY, RELIGION, AND HEALTH

Many cultures of the world believe that spirituality and health are intimately connected. In *Ageless Body, Timeless Mind*, Dr. Deepak Chopra (1993) explains the interconnectedness of mind, body, and spirit this way: "Spirituality is not meant to be separate from the body... Sickness and aging represent the body's inability to reach its natural goal, which is to join the mind in perfection and fulfillment" (p. 167).

Since the energy force of spirituality is often transmitted through religious practices that can provide both the health care provider and the individual with insight, meaning, and healing, it's easy to see that complex connections exist between spiritual and religious beliefs and practices and an individual's physical and psychological health. Long before antibiotics, aspirin, extracts, or x-rays, people who were ill turned to spiritual or religious healers to help them get better. Religious and spiritual concerns with health and illness date back to the beginning of human history. For example, as early as 100,000 years ago, humans began using rituals when burying their dead, presumably to provide for their well-being in another life (O'Hara, 2002). While modern Western medicine has increasingly focused on the physiologic aspects of disease and on technology for cures, many individuals and health care providers now focus on the whole person, including the spiritual dimension.

Medical, social science, and psychological literature all support the positive link between spirituality, religion, and health. The supportive community and meaningful life of a spiritual and/or religious individual mean better health, lower mortality, and less disease. Religious beliefs and practices, such as prayer, trusting in

God, turning problems over to God, and support from a minister or congregation, become extremely important to people when they become physically ill and must face the possibilities of surgery or rehabilitation. Religious beliefs become stronger as a result of these stressors (Koenig, 2000).

Religious participation also increases with increasing age. Whether this is because older persons today were raised during a time when religion was very important or because religious people tend to live longer is not known, but many older adults state that religion is the most important factor in helping them cope with a physical illness or life stressor or adapting to personal losses or the difficulties of caregiving (Ebersole & Hess, 1997; Koenig, 2000).

According to Skokan and Bader (2000), spirituality can bring an ill person three benefits: hope, strength, and emotional support. As a result, spiritual individuals can experience a sense of satisfaction with their lives even in the face of illness. Koenig (1999) also refers to another benefit of spirituality—spiritual joy. Spiritual joy is an intense, personally satisfying experience that goes beyond loving friendship to a transcendental experience. This joy can exert a powerful influence in the individual's participation in life-enhancing, life-promoting activities.

Research Findings

While participation in religious activities is, perhaps, the easiest way to measure religiosity, many studies have uncovered the powerful connection between spirituality, religion, and health (Larson, Swyers, & McCullough, 1998; Matthews & Clark, 1998). For example, scientific studies show that religious involvement "helps people *prevent* illness, *recover* from illness, and—most remarkably—*live longer*" (Matthews & Clark, 1998, p. 19).

According to Matthews & Clark (1998), research has shown that those who attend religious services one or more times a week have dramatically lower death rates than their counterparts who do not attend religious services as frequently. Deaths from coronary artery disease showed a 50% reduction, emphysema showed a 56% reduction, cirrhosis of the liver showed a 74% reduction, and suicide was reduced by 53%. Certain sexually transmitted diseases, pulmonary tuberculosis, and abnormal cervical cytologies were also reduced.

Other research on the connection between religion and health since that time has demonstrated the following:

- There is a positive relationship between religion and physical, as well as mental, health (Astedt-Kurki, 1995; Ebersole & Hess, 1997; Koenig, 1999, 2000; Levin et al., 1996).
- Persons who attend religious services regularly (once a week or more) are only about half as likely to be depressed as those who do not attend services (Koenig, George, & Peterson, 1998; Mueller et al., 2001).
- Many people depend on religion and spirituality as their primary method of coping with physical health problems and the stress of surgery (Boudreaux et al., 2002; Koenig, 2000).
- Religiousness may alter the perception of disability such that those who are more religious actually perceive themselves as less disabled and more physically capable than those who are less religious (Koenig, 2000).
- Adults who both attend weekly religious services and read religious scriptures at least daily are less likely to experience high blood pressure (Koenig, George, Cohen, et al., 1998a; Larson & Koenig, 2000; Mueller et al., 2001).

- Higher levels of religious involvement are associated with the practice of positive health-related behaviors such as self-care and hygienic regimens (Koenig, 2000; Levin et al., 1996).
- Most older persons report that religion helps them to cope with or adapt to personal losses or difficulties, such as caregiving (Ebersole & Hess, 1997; Koenig, 2000).
- Adults who both attend weekly religious services and pray or read religious scriptures daily are almost 90% less likely to smoke cigarettes. Many are less likely to begin smoking (Koenig, 2000; Koenig, George, Cohen, et al., 1998b).
- People with strong spiritual beliefs seem to resolve their grief more rapidly and completely after the death of a close person than do people with no spiritual beliefs (Walsh, King, Jones, Tookman, & Blizard, 2002).
- Religious attendance has been associated with a longer life, more hopefulness, less depression, healthier lifestyle choices, longer marriages, and an expanded social network (Koenig, 2000; Koenig et al., 1999; Larson & Koenig, 2000; Westlake, 2001).
- Religious involvement may help boost immune system functioning, facilitate healing and recovery, and prevent infection after surgery (Koenig, 1999, 2000).
- Religious involvement is associated with less cardiovascular disease and cardiovascular mortality (Koenig, 1999; Mueller et al., 2001) and a decreased incidence of cancer (Mull, Cox, & Sullivan, 1987).

Although research has demonstrated that participation in religious activities is an important component in preventing disease, achieving a state of well-being, healing from illness, and extending the life span, one mystery remains: why some people are cured and others are not. It is important to remember that religious participation and spirituality are no guarantee for physical health (Matthews & Clark, 1998).

Religion and Negative Health Effects

Not all of the evidence is conclusive, but some research supports the view that religious affiliation can have negative consequences on an individual's health and well-being (Koenig, 2000; Mueller et al., 2001; O'Hara, 2002). Koenig (2000) and Mueller et al. (2001) list the following negative consequences:

- Devout religiousness may cause excessive guilt, narrow-mindedness, and inflexibility that may lead to neuroses.
- Religious cults can isolate and alienate individuals from their family, friends, and community and may even encourage self-destruction (e.g., Reverend Jim Jones' group in Jonestown, Guyana).
- Some religious groups may discourage appropriate mental and physical health care or encourage the discontinuance of traditional treatments.
- Some religious beliefs may support the failure to seek timely medical care or discourage effective preventive health measures (such as childhood immunizations and prenatal care).
- Religiously involved persons may have unrealistically high expectations for themselves, resulting in anxiety, isolation, alienation, or depression.
- Religious preoccupations and delusions are often a component of obsessive-compulsive, manic-depressive, and schizophrenic individuals.

THE BENEFITS OF RELIGION ON SPECIFIC HEALTH CONDITIONS

Individuals with life-threatening or chronic health conditions can benefit greatly from spirituality and religious practices. Individuals with cancer, asthma, human immunodeficiency virus (HIV), chronic pain, multiple sclerosis, burns, end-stage renal disease, and coronary artery disease all report that religious and spiritual beliefs and practices help them cope with their disease (Mueller et al., 2001). Since spirituality involves finding meaning in life and its experiences, the seriously or chronically ill person must actively engage in the process of "finding" that meaning (Skokan & Bader, 2000).

A great deal of current knowledge about the connection between spirituality, religion, and health has come from studies examining cancer, since a diagnosis of cancer often raises deep spiritual issues (Boudreaux et al., 2002). Although further research is needed, a link between spirituality, religion, and health has been established:

- Religious beliefs had a positive impact on spiritual well-being in women with breast cancer (Mickley et al., 1992).
- Spirituality and presence are believed to play crucial roles in an individual's recovery from acute illness and surgery and from an acute myocardial infarction (Boudreaux et al., 2002; Walton, 1999).
- Spirituality seems to improve resiliency, well-being, and the ability to cope with difficult life events in those people with HIV/AIDS. Distance healing and intercessory prayer has been effective in wound healing (Boudreaux et al., 2002; Coward, 1995; Koenig et al., 1997).
- Individuals with rheumatoid arthritis derived significant short- and long-term physical benefits from in-person intercessory prayer ministry (Matthews, 2000)
- Religious activities have enhanced people's ability to cope with many chronic illnesses, including cystic fibrosis, diabetes, chronic renal failure, coronary artery disease, and spinal cord injury (Matthews, 2000).
- End-of-life care emphasizes the physical and spiritual aspect of care. Many terminally ill individuals derive great strength and hope from their religious and spiritual beliefs (Mueller et al., 2001).

RELIGIOUS BELIEFS, RELIGIOUS PRACTICES, AND HEALTH

As immigrants have come to America, they have brought with them the world's religious traditions—Buddhism, Hinduism, Islam, Judaism, and Christianity, among many others. As a result, the United States is the most religiously diverse nation on the earth (Eck, 2001).

The many diverse religious faiths that make up the United States often come to mind when health care providers think about the spiritual aspect of care. This religious diversity impacts health and the delivery of health care. According to Rhi (2001), "Religious cultures are the most powerful factors that modify the individual's attitudes toward life, death, happiness, and suffering" (p. 573). They influence every aspect of mental and physical health, to varying degrees.

Since a person's religious beliefs influence how he or she interprets life experiences, personal health, illness, and death, providing spiritually-appropriate care means becoming familiar with religious beliefs and practices. Health care is provided more effectively when professionals have at least some knowledge of the various major religious traditions that influence client attitudes toward health and health care (Taylor, 2002). The relationship between an individual's religion and culture should also be evaluated in-depth, since one might, for example, encounter a Korean client who identifies himself as a Protestant but occasionally consults a fortuneteller and also participates in Confucian ancestor worship (Rhi, 2001).

While Western health care providers often come from a primarily Judeo-Christian background, a broader understanding of other faiths and perspectives is important. To assist health care professionals in understanding and appreciating the similarities among major world religions, especially with regard to the health care practices and rituals specific to each, this section briefly describes the religious traditions and health care practices of some of the most commonly seen religions in the United States: Buddhism, Hinduism, Islam, Judaism, and Christianity.

Please note: This section is not meant to serve as an in-depth examination of all the world's religions, nor is it intended to stereotype individuals or their religions in any way. It is simply offered as an overview to help broaden the health care provider's and spiritual care provider's awareness and allow them to provide spiritually compassionate care.

Buddhism

Many schools of thought and many sects exist within the Buddhist religion (Northcott, 2002). However, certain core beliefs unify this religion. Buddhism does not recognize a single supreme, personalized being whose word must be followed. It recognizes, rather, an accumulation of wisdom to which each generation adds its understandings.

Approximately 2,500 years ago, a prince was born who became known as Buddha, the Enlightened One, or the Awakened Being. Buddhism teaches that Buddha can show the way to enlightenment, but it is up to each person to practice a way of life that emphasizes compassion, mind control, transformation of negative thought, and attainment of ultimate wisdom (Eck, 2001; Hitchcock, Schubert, & Thomas, 1999; Taylor, 2002).

Buddhists believe in the theory of karma (i.e., for every action there is a consequence, and the consequence will occur either in this life or a future life) (Eck, 2001; Hitchcock et al., 1999; Taylor, 2002). The primary religious goal of Buddhism is to achieve the state of One-Mind (*Il-shim*) or nirvana, a state of liberation that follows the concepts of divine teachings and a peaceful, harmonious existence of humility (Northcott, 2002; Rhi, 2001).

Health beliefs and practices are synonymous in Buddhism and include the following (Hitchcock et al., 1999; Taylor, 2002):
- Meditation and mind control
- Chanting
- The four requisites (proper clothing, food, lodging, and medicine)
- Vegetarianism
- Avoidance of alcohol and tobacco

- Emetics and purging
- Oils and ointments
- Medicinal drugs and herbs
- Surgery

In addition, Buddhism holds the belief of continual rebirth, or reincarnation, until nirvana or liberation is experienced. Buddhism places a high value on compassion. Organ donation, for example, is not strictly prohibited (Gillman, 1999).

Inn and *ko* (cause and effect) are principles of Buddhism that encourage people to "do the right thing" and receive good in return. In Buddhism, fate, inn, and ko are the main factors that determine health. When people are aware of their behavior and are morally good, they have little guilt, peace of mind, and health and well-being (Chen, 2001).

Hinduism

Hinduism is believed to be the oldest of the world's religions, dating from about 2500 BC. Derived from the name of the river in India now called Indus, Hinduism is a fusion of traditions and shared beliefs (Jootun, 2002). It reflects a metaphysical understanding and way of life that defines morals, customs, medicine, art, music, and dance. The one major guiding philosophy for all Hindus is that all is Brahman, the Supreme Being.

Health practices in the Hindu culture are based on an understanding of prana, the life force energy of humans. In Hinduism, chakras (energy centers) are associated with consciousness and with body functions. When these primary forces are in harmony, good health results. When there is disharmony, disease or illness is thought to result (Hitchcock et al., 1999; Taylor, 2002).

Hinduism's customs, beliefs, and values are based on the assumption that every living thing has a soul that passes through successive cycles of birth and rebirth. The Hindu idea of karma is that each person is reborn so "the soul may be purified and ultimately join the divine cosmic consciousness" (Jootun, 2002, p. 38). Hinduism views the person as a combination of mind, body, and soul within a context of family, culture, and environment. Purity is important (Jootun, 2002).

In Hinduism, disease is a reflection of the individual's life. Therefore, the person's diet, relationships, personal thoughts, attitudes, and lifestyle along with the environment and the seasons are considered when treating or diagnosing a client. Treatment focuses on balancing "the humors" (i.e., air, fire, earth, and water). Balancing these humors and releasing toxins by means of diet, fasting, enemas, purgatives, and massage are the goals of treatment. Rituals often include the use of fire, water, light, scents, sounds, flowers, postures, gestures, and mantras. Many Hindus are vegetarians for spiritual reasons. They do not eat beef and pork because they view the cow as a sacred animal and the pig as a scavenger whose meat is "dirty." The Hindu religious calendar includes numerous festivals, fasts, and holidays (Hitchcock et al., 1999; Jootun, 2002; Taylor, 2002).

Islam

Islam has its roots in seventh-century Arabia, although Islam is not an "Arabic" religion (Hedayat & Pirzadeh, 2001). The Arabic word *Islam* means submission and is derived from a word meaning peace. Islam is a sociology and philosophy for life and includes a belief in holism. The followers of Islam are known as Muslims. Today, there are approximately 1.3 billion Muslims in the world (Rassool, 2000).

Around 570 AD, the prophet Muhammad was born. The Koran (the sacred book of Islam) records the teachings that were channeled through Muhammad by the archangel Gabriel while Muhammad prayed in a cave. Among those teachings, the nature of God as the Absolute was made known. *Allah*, the Arabic name for God, is the term used by Arabic Muslims and Christians as well as non-Arab Muslims.

The Koran says there is no God but Allah and warns against the worship of idols (Hitchcock et al., 1999). Islam's main tenet is, "There is no God but Allah, and Muhammad is His messenger" (Taylor, 2002, p. 237). The Koran is placed above all other books (literally and philosophically) and so it is never to be placed on the floor (Akhtar, 2002).

In Islam, human beings are the "crown of creation" (Daar & Al Khitamy, 2001, p. 61). Duties and obligations are extremely important. Children are valued and respected in Islam as individuals with inherent rights, including the right to be respected and not treated violently. The mother's role is to raise morally and physically sound children, while the father is responsible for education, marriage, and all financial costs related to child-rearing (Hedayat & Pirzadeh, 2001).

The "Five Pillars of Faith" are Islamic religious rituals and practices and include the following (Akhtar, 2002; Hitchcock et al., 1999; Rassool, 2000; Taylor, 2002):

1. **Profession of faith:** There is no God but Allah, and Muhammad is His messenger. This first article of faith is called the Shahadah.
2. **Prayer:** Obligatory prayers are performed five times a day while facing the city of Mecca (at dawn, midday, late afternoon, sunset, and late evening).
3. **Almsgiving:** Giving alms or charity (called Zakat) is a form of purification and growth. Wealth is purified by setting aside a proportion for others in need.
4. **Fasting:** Fasting is regarded as a spiritual means of self-purification and involves prayer, reflection, and positive thoughts toward others. Daily fasting from dawn to sunset during the month of Ramadan means abstaining from eating, drinking, and sexual relations. Children begin fasting and praying when they reach puberty.
5. **Pilgrimage:** Making a pilgrimage to Mecca (called Hajj) in the Kingdom of Saudi Arabia should happen at least once in a person's lifetime, if possible. Individuals who make the pilgrimage wear simple clothing so status, class, culture, and color are not disclosed, and all are equal before Allah.

Five goals for believers of Islam include protecting life, mind, religion, family, and property (Taylor, 2002). Thus, for those who practice Islam, a health care decision may be influenced by the goal of protecting life.

While Muslims may consider illness an atonement for their sins, they do not consider it a punishment or an expression of Allah's wrath (Daar & Al Khitamy, 2001). Muslims view death as part of a journey to meet their God. They believe health and illness are part of a continuum of being, and they receive illness and death with patience, meditation, and prayers (Rassool, 2000). According to Rassool (2000), other Islamic health practices include the following:

- Regard for the sanctity of life
- Moderate eating
- Regular exercise, prayers, fasting, and bathing
- Abstinence from alcohol, tobacco, and other psychoactive substances

- Circumcisions of male infants
- Blood transfusions after proper screening
- No autopsies, abortions (except to save a mother's life), assisted suicide, or euthanasia
- Transplantation of organs (with some restrictions)
- Prohibition of homosexuality (but caring for individuals with AIDS)

Caring is embedded in the framework of Islam. Allah expects human beings to care for the weak. Spiritual care is important, and respect for diversity and tolerance of non-Muslim individuals is expected.

Judaism

Judaism is best understood through the history of the Jewish people, a group of ethnically, socially, and culturally diverse people. There are an estimated 10 million Jewish people in the world (Collins, 2002). However, not all Jews practice Judaism.

Judaism has three main branches: Orthodox, Conservative, and Reform. Judaism holds that the saving of a human life takes precedence over all other laws and is believed to be the noblest act a person can perform. Thus, organ donation is an acceptable act to many Jews (Gillman, 1999).

The Jewish people who practice Judaism have a highly moral lifestyle that regards the Torah and its commandments and teachings as a guide for a way of life (Collins, 2002). Teachings of Judaism include the following (Hitchcock et al., 1999):

- The divine covenant with God can never be broken.
- The law as set forth in the Bible as the Ten Commandments must always be followed.
- God has promised a vision of a new heaven and a new Earth with the coming of the Messiah.
- There is only one God.
- Only the sins of humankind separate people from the divine.
- The Sabbath is the central day of the week.
- Humans are to love, praise, and serve God above all else.
- The Torah (the five books of Moses) holds Judaism's laws and sacred traditions.
- The family is seen as the basic unit of society and has sacred obligations to maintain integrity and purity in relationship with God.
- Spirit and body are considered separated at death.

Certain Judaic practices involve laws governing food types that cannot be eaten (such as pork, shellfish, and their derivatives) and the utensils in which food may be cooked. Meat, milk, and milk products may not be eaten together or cooked together (Collins, 2002).

Christianity

With the birth of Jesus Christ in Palestine during the reign of Herod the Great, Christianity emerged. Christianity teaches of one God consisting of a trinity—Father, Son, and Holy Spirit.

Christianity is found in almost every country in the world and includes three major branches: Catholics, Protestants, and Orthodox. Christianity is made up of many denominations or churches, with each having its own set of beliefs, practices, and rituals (Eck, 2001; Hitchcock et al., 1999; Taylor, 2002). These include the Church of England, Catholicism, Orthodox Christianity, Presbyterianism, Methodism, Pentecostalism, Seventh Day Adventism, as well as many others (Christmas, 2002). Christians use the Bible as the source of inspiration; however, interpretations may vary.

The primary goal of Christianity is salvation (Rhi, 2001). Those who live a good Christian life will go to heaven and be with Jesus Christ (Christmas, 2002). According to orthodox Christian religions, such as Greek Orthodox, all people should be treated with respect and dignity. Home and family life are central to the orthodox lifestyle (Papadopoulos, 2002).

The use of prayer is common to all denominations. Christians hold different views on what happens after a person dies, but they generally accept that there is an afterlife and that God's final judgment determines an individual's ultimate future of heaven or hell. Two rituals that are practiced include *communion*, the ingestion of bread and wine as symbols of Jesus' body and blood, and *baptism*, an immersion in or application of water to signify cleansing from sin and passage into Christianity (Eck, 2001; Hitchcock et al., 1999; Taylor, 2002).

Health beliefs and practices vary widely among each of the three branches of Christianity. The Bible includes many examples of Jesus healing the sick through laying on of hands, faith healing, and releasing demons. Specific practices, such as organ donation, also vary. For example, Protestant Christians are in favor of organ donation, while Jehovah's Witnesses support organ donation only as long as all blood is removed from the organs and tissues before they are transplanted (Gillman, 1999).

Judeo-Christian Beliefs

Since Western health care providers often come from a primarily Judeo-Christian background, an examination of their common beliefs may be helpful. According to Matthews & Clark (1998), the Judeo-Christian perspective shares the following beliefs:

- God is seen as a person to whom human beings can relate as a person.
- While human beings are made in the image of God, He is transcendent, omnipotent, omnipresent, and far greater than humans can imagine.
- There is a moral code to be obeyed, and while there are different interpretations of this code, people strive to know God's will and live by it.
- God has given humans free will. While He acts in their lives, they can choose to accept or reject Him.

INTEGRATING RELIGIOUS PRACTICES AND BELIEFS INTO HEALTH CARE

To provide spiritually compassionate care, health care professionals need to consider both religious and spiritual needs when planning care for their clients. Rules regarding right and wrong as well as guidelines for handling these issues are usually included in religious teachings. However, health care professionals need to be aware of the diversity of religious practices that exist both within and between faiths, as well as the various spiritual beliefs. Because religious beliefs originate from a particular worldview, rules and values may vary among different religions or cultures. For example, Orthodox Muslim women have very strict rules for proper public dress but not all Muslim women will follow those rules.

Caution should be exercised in planning care. Just because someone belongs to a particular faith does not mean he or she actively practices that faith. For example, some Catholic clients may not wish to have a priest called to tend to their spiritual needs. Health care professionals should always ask clients or their families about their specific spiritual needs before intervening (Burkhardt & Nathaniel, 1998).

SUMMARY

Religion is the practical expression of spirituality and involves the organization, rituals, and practice of one's spiritual beliefs. This practical expression can be a powerful healing force when it is transmitted between the knowledgeable, compassionate health care provider and the client. While a few aspects of religion may have some negative effects on the well-being of some individuals, it provides most with tremendous benefits.

KEY CONCEPTS

1. *Spirituality* is a broader concept than religion and is primarily a dynamic, personal, and experiential process. *Religion* is usually recognized as the practical expression of spirituality (i.e., the organization, rituals, and practice of one's beliefs).
2. Religious and spiritual concerns with health and illness date back to the beginning of human history.
3. While religion and spirituality are not "magic bullets" that prevent aging, illness, and disease, the medical, social science, and psychological literature support a positive link between religion, spirituality, and health. However, religion and spirituality may also have some negative effects on an individual's health and well-being.
4. Health care is provided more effectively when professionals have at least some knowledge of the various religious traditions that influence client attitudes toward health and health care.
5. Both the nonreligious client and the nonreligious health care provider may still consider themselves spiritual. Supportive care can be provided regardless of whether an individual is an agnostic, an atheist, or a religious follower.

QUESTIONS FOR REFLECTION

1. Caring for the "whole person" includes paying attention to and nurturing the person's religious and/or spiritual needs. Sometimes, a health care provider's own views can get in the way of providing compassionate care. Take a moment to reflect upon your views and any ways in which they may interfere with your ability to provide care. If you are nonreligious, do you sometimes overlook the importance of religion to others? If you are extremely religious, do you have difficulty relating to someone who disagrees with your views?

2. Your patient or client asks you to pray with her, but you know your religion and religious beliefs are quite different from hers. What do you do?

REFERENCES

Akhtar, S. G. (2002). Nursing with dignity, part 8: Islam. *Nursing Times, 98*(16), 40-42.

Astedt-Kurki, P. (1995). Religiosity as a dimension of well-being. *Clinical Nursing Research, 4*(4), 387-397.

Boudreaux, E. D., O'Hea, E., & Chasuk, R. (2002). Spiritual role in healing: An alternative way of thinking. *Primary Care: Clinics in Office Practice, 29*(2), viii, 439-454.

Burkhardt, M. A., & Nathaniel, A. K. (1998). *Ethics and issues.* New York: Delmar.

Chen, Y. C. (2001). Chinese values, health, and nursing. *Journal of Advanced Nursing, 36*(2), 270-273.

Chopra, D. (1993). *Ageless body, timeless mind.* New York: Harmony Books.

Christmas, M. (2002). Nursing with dignity, part 3: Christianity I. *Nursing Times, 98*(11), 37-39.

Collins, A. (2002). Nursing with dignity, part 1: Judaism. *Nursing Times, 98*(9), 34-35.

Coward, D. D. (1995). The lived experience of self-transcendence in women with AIDS. *Journal of Obstetric, Gynecologic, and Neonatal Nurses, 24*(4), 314-318.

Coyle, J. (2002). Spirituality and health: Towards a framework for exploring the relationship. *Journal of Advanced Nursing, 37*(6), 589-597.

Daar, A. S., & Al Khitamy, A. B. (2001). Bioethics for clinicians: 21. Islamic bioethics. *Canadian Medical Association Journal, 164*(1), 60-63.

Dossey, L. (1993). *Healing words: The power of prayer and the practice of medicine.* San Francisco: HarperCollins.

Dossey, L. (1996). *Prayer is good medicine.* San Francisco: HarperCollins.

Ebersole, P., & Hess, P. (1997). *Toward healthy aging: Human needs and nursing response* (5th ed.). St. Louis, MO: Mosby-Year Book.

Eck, D. (2001). *A new religious America.* San Francisco: HarperCollins.

Gillman, J. (1999). Religious perspectives on organ donation. *Critical Care Nursing Quarterly, 22*(3), 19-29.

Goddard, N. (2000). A response to Dawson's critical analysis of "spirituality as 'integrative energy.'" *Journal of Advanced Nursing, 31*(4), 968-979.

Hedayat, K. M., & Pirzadeh, R. (2001). Issues in Islamic biomedical ethics: A primer for the pediatrician. *Pediatrics, 108*(4), 965-971.

Hitchcock, J. E., Schubert, P. E., & Thomas, S. A. (1999). *Community health nursing: Caring in action.* Albany, NY: Delmar Thomson Learning.

Jootun, D. (2002). Nursing with dignity, part 7: Hinduism. *Nursing Times, 98*(13), 38-40.

Koenig, H. G. (1999). *The healing power of faith.* New York: Simon & Schuster.

Koenig, H. G. (2000). Spiritual aspects of surgery. *Ophthalmology Clinics of North America, 13*(1), 71-83.

Koenig, H. G., Cohen, H. J., George, L. K., Hays, J. C., Larson, D. B., & Blazer, D. G. (1997). Attendance at religious services, interleukin-6, and other biological parameters of immune function in older adults. *International Journal of Psychiatry in Medicine, 27*(3), 233-250.

Koenig, H. G., George, L. K., Cohen, H. J., Hays, J. C., Larson, D. B., & Blazer, D. G. (1998a). The relationship between religious activities and blood pressure in older adults. *International Journal of Psychiatry in Medicine, 28*(2), 189-213.

Koenig, H. G., George, L. K., Cohen, H. J., Hays, J. C., Larson, D. B., & Blazer, D. G. (1998b). The relationship between religious activities and cigarette smoking in older adults. *Journal of Gerontology: Medical Sciences, 53A*(6), M426-M434.

Koenig, H. G., George, L. K., & Peterson, B. L. (1998). Religiosity and remission of depression in medically ill older patients. *American Journal of Psychiatry, 155*(4), 536-542.

Koenig, H. G., Hays, J. C., Larson, D. B., George, L. K., Cohen, H. J., McCullough, M. E., et al. (1999). Does religious attendance prolong survival? A six-year follow-up study of 3,968 older adults. *Journal of Gerontology: Medical Sciences, 54A*(7), M370-M376.

Larson, D. B., & Koenig, H. G. (2000). Is God good for your health? The role of spirituality in medical care. *Cleveland Clinic Journal of Medicine, 67*(2), 80-84.

Larson, D. B., Swyers, J. P., & McCullough, M. E. (1998). *Scientific research on spirituality and health.* Rockville, MD: National Institute for Healthcare Research.

Levin, J. S., Chatters, L. M., Ellison, C. G., & Taylor, R. J. (1996). Religious involvement, health outcomes, and public health practice. *Current Issues in Public Health, 2,* 220-225.

Macrae, J. A. (2001). *Nursing as a spiritual practice.* New York: Springer.

Matthews, D. A. (2000). Prayer and spirituality. *Rheumatic Diseases Clinics of North America, 26*(1), xi, 177-187.

Matthews, D. A., & Clark, C. (1998). *The faith factor: Proof of the healing power of prayer.* New York: Penguin Books.

Mickley, J. R., Soeken, K., & Belcher, A. (1992). Spiritual well-being, religiousness, and hope among women with breast cancer. *Image: Journal of Nursing Scholarship, 24*(4), 267-272.

Mueller, P. S., Plevak, D. J., & Rummans, T. A. (2001). Religious involvement, spirituality, and medicine: Implications for clinical practice. *Mayo Clinic Proceedings, 76*(12), 1225-1235.

Mull, C. S., Cox, C. L., & Sullivan, J. A. (1987). Religion's role in the health and well-being of well elders. *Public Health Nursing, 4*(3), 151-159.

Narayanasamy, A. (1999). A review of spirituality as applied to nursing. *International Journal of Nursing Studies, 36,* 117-125.

Northcott, N. (2002). Nursing with dignity, part 2: Buddhism. *Nursing Times, 98*(10), 36-38.

O'Hara, D. P. (2002). Is there a role for prayer and spirituality in health care? *Medical Clinics of North America, 86*(1), vi, 33-46.

Papadopoulos, I. (2002). Nursing with dignity, part 4: Christianity II. *Nursing Times, 98*(12), 36-37.

Rassool, G. H. (2000). The crescent and Islam: Healing, nursing, and the spiritual dimension. Some considerations toward an understanding of the Islamic perspectives of caring. *Journal of Advanced Nursing, 32*(6), 1476-1484.

Rhi, B.Y. (2001). Culture, spirituality, and mental health: The forgotten aspects of religion and health. *Psychiatric Clinics of North America, 24*(3), ix-x, 569-579.

Scott, R. O. (2001). A look in the mirror: Finding our way in this new spiritual landscape. *Spirituality and Aging, 4*(1), 26.

Skokan, L., & Bader, D. (2000). Spirituality and healing. *Health Progress, 81*(1), 38-42.

Taylor, E. J. (2002). *Spiritual care.* Upper Saddle River, NJ: Prentice Hall.

Walsh, K., King, M., Jones, L., Tookman, A., & Blizard, R. (2002). Spiritual beliefs may affect outcome of bereavement: Prospective study. *British Journal of Medicine, 324*(7353), 1551.

Walton, J. (1999). Spirituality of patients recovering from an acute myocardial infarction: A grounded theory study. *Journal of Holistic Nursing, 17*(1), 34-53.

Westlake, C. (2001). Role of spirituality in adjustment of patients with advanced heart disease. *Progressive Cardiovascular Nursing, 16*(3), 119-125.

5

SPIRITUALITY, CULTURE, AND HEALTH

"A Navajo weaver takes strands of wool and blends them into something of great beauty and magic; warp and weft combine into a pattern, and the pattern tells a story and has a spirit. This pattern then becomes a piece of the culture and has a life of its own. From the beginning I knew I had to do a similar thing with the strands of my story—to tell how a girl from a small and remote town on an Indian reservation was able to become a surgeon, able to work in the high-tech realm of a surgical operating room, and combine that with another story, about how ancient tribal ways and philosophies can help a floundering medical system find its way back to its original mission: healing."
—Lori Arviso Alvord, MD, First female Navajo surgeon
(Alvord & Van Pelt, 1999)

LEARNING OBJECTIVES

Upon completing this chapter, you will be able to do the following:
1. Describe the relationship between spirituality, culture, and health.
2. Define *compassion* and explain what is meant by culturally competent care.
3. Examine the components of a cultural and spiritual self-assessment.
4. Identify three major health belief systems.
5. Identify four major health care systems.
6. Describe specific characteristics about the composition, spiritual and religious practices, cultural aspects, and unique health care issues of African Americans, Asian Americans, Hispanic Americans, Native Americans, and Arab Americans.
7. Explain the relationship between language and culturally competent care.

INTRODUCTION

Until the end of the medieval period, religion, spirituality, and medicine remained integrated in the West. Monasteries housed the first hospitals, and physicians were commonly monks. As Matthews (1999) explains, "At one time, medicine and religion were so thoroughly united that a medicine man was a priest. Many cultures throughout the world still regard their healer in just this way" (p. 17). However, medicine, spirituality, culture, and religion became separated during the scientific revolution. For many years, spiritual care fell into disuse.

Today, emerging scientific evidence demonstrates the connection between religion, spirituality, and health (Matthews, 1999). With the increasing movement toward holistic care and a multicultural society, competent health care professionals need to integrate cultural as well as spiritual sensitivity into their clients' health care considerations.

While all people are equal and deserve to be treated with kindness, dignity, and respect, all people do not share the same values, beliefs, and cultural backgrounds. The United States demonstrates the truth of this statement through its unique blending of native and nonnative peoples. In addition, because of advancements in technology, travel, and communication systems, people of many different cultures enjoy increased contact with each other (Hitchcock, Schubert, & Thomas, 1999). Today's health care professionals are presented with the challenge of providing a level of care that respects different cultural values and cultural belief systems. Meeting these varied needs in a multicultural society is an essential part of health care. Understanding and respecting diverse cultural populations and their spiritual beliefs allows health care professionals to effectively address the special health concerns of their clients and is an important part of providing culturally competent, effective clinical and spiritual care.

The provision of health care needs to encompass a more holistic perspective—one that attends to all aspects of the mind, body, and spirit. Health care professionals who understand the importance of integrating cultural sensitivity with spirituality can provide more efficient and higher quality care (Davidhizar, Bechtel, & Juratovac, 2000).

CULTURE DEFINED

Bonder, Martin, and Miracle (2002) in *Culture in Clinical Care*, define culture as:
- Learned: By listening to, observing, and assessing interactions with others.
- Localized: By interactions in personally meaningful locales in multiple social settings with specific individuals.
- Patterned: Through the repetition of specific samples of behavior and talk.
- Evaluative: By the reflection of cultural values in individual behavioral decisions and choices.
- Persistent: By being stable but also incorporating change as the individual experiences new objects, situations, and ideas over the life course.

Culture can be learned from birth through language and socialization; it is dynamic and changing, and it continually adapts to the environment, social and historical context, technology, and resources. Culture is generally unexpressed and rarely discussed at a conscious level. Most cultural actions are based on implicit cues instead of written or spoken rules. Culture is "a universal phenomenon that is learned and transmitted from one generation to another, providing the blueprint for a person's beliefs, behaviors, attitudes, and values" (Lueckenotte, 1996, p. 134).

In the United States, individuals of diverse cultural backgrounds create a rainbow of color and culture. This country's diverse population and the resulting cultural mix result from many factors, including the following (Bonder et al., 2002; Dossey, Keegan, & Guzzetta, 2000):

- The climate, food availability, and resources of a particular area.
- Migration patterns determined by climate, environmental conditions, and political and economic situations (e.g., famine, political uprising, war, epidemics, or overpopulation).
- Changing social roles of women.
- Changing value orientations and beliefs (including changes in beliefs about humanity's relationship to nature and to other persons).
- Technological innovations.
- Communication patterns and methods.
- Diverse health care beliefs.

Most people in this country don't wake up in the morning and say, "I'm an African American," or "I'm an Asian American." If anything, they probably say, "I'm an American." However, Americans stem from an incredible array of cultural backgrounds, and that factor plays an important role in every aspect of an individual's life.

HOW ARE SPIRITUALITY, CULTURE, AND HEALTH RELATED?

Earlier chapters of this book described the impact of spirituality on health and health behaviors. Like spirituality, culture also has a significant impact on health behaviors; health problems; and actions taken to promote, maintain, or restore health. Because spirituality and culture play an important role in health and healing, health care providers need to understand how these concepts intertwine.

- **Healing** is a spiritual process that attends to the wholeness of a person (i.e., mind-body-spirit) (Burkhardt & Nagai-Jacobson, 2002). Within cultures, healing has been closely linked to understanding the sacred and the spiritual. Burkhardt and Nagai-Jacobson (2002) state, "The resurgence of a holistic view of persons among conventional health care practitioners, coupled with exposure to views of sickness and healing within explanatory models from different cultures and traditions, have contributed to this awareness" (p. 26).
- **Spirituality** is an integral part of the health, healing, and well-being of every individual. It is expressed and experienced through an interconnectedness with nature, the earth, the environment, the cosmos, and other people. In other words, spirituality is intertwined with every aspect of life and provides purpose, meaning, strength, and guidance in shaping the journey of life.
- **Culture** is "the whole of ideas, customs, skills, arts, and other capabilities of a people or group, although as a whole, it is more complex than any one of these elements" (Dossey et al., 2000, p. 284). Culture helps people define who they are and what they believe; it influences the way they address life, death, birth,

childbearing, child rearing, illness, disease, dietary habits, relationships, and health behaviors (Hitchcock et al., 1999). Culture also impacts the delivery of health care services, the understanding of disease and illness, and the way care is provided.

The values and beliefs of a culture are determined in part by spirituality and religion, which play a prominent role in how people interpret, make sense of, and cope with an illness (Taylor, 2002). In addition, culture determines how people view and make sense of the world and how they experience health, illness, and medical care. Cultural beliefs and rituals help clients and their families cope with stress, fear, and illness. Cultural differences may cause misunderstandings among clients and health care providers.

Martsolf (1997) suggests three ways in which spirituality and culture are related:
1. Spirituality can be determined entirely by culture.
2. Spirituality can be determined by life experiences unrelated to culture.
3. Spirituality can be influenced by both culture and personal experiences that are in opposition to the cultural norm.

Culture includes spirituality and religious practices, which are intimately related to health beliefs and practices, and ultimately to health and healing. Since spirituality and culture affect all dimensions of an individual's health and healing, the health care professional or spiritual care provider should carefully consider them when planning and delivering culturally sensitive, compassionate, competent care.

COMPASSION AND CULTURALLY COMPETENT CARE

Compassion as a spiritual quality resides at the heart of culturally competent care. The word *compassion* comes from the Latin *compassio*, which means "to feel with." Discovered by both mystics and scientists, compassion is the ultimate unity of life. It involves a respect for the self as well as for others. Embracing all individuals regardless of culture, personal attributes, or religion, compassion can be viewed as a spiritual or universal love (Macrae, 2001).

Culturally competent care is not limited to but can involve the following (Leininger & McFarland, 2002):
- An awareness of one's own experience, thoughts, beliefs, and values without the biased influence of those from other cultures.
- Knowledge and understanding of the client's culture.
- A respect and acceptance of cultural differences.
- An adaptation of care that is congruent with the client's culture.

A lack of respect for persons of differing cultural values can lead to potential and real harm, either culturally, psychologically, physically, or spiritually. Conversely, the delivery of culturally and spiritually competent care leads to improved health outcomes, increased efficiency in the delivery of services, and increased client satisfaction.

LOOKING WITHIN:
A SPIRITUAL AND CULTURAL SELF-ASSESSMENT

One way health care providers can discover and better understand their clients' spiritual and cultural beliefs and practices is to conduct a self-assessment of their own spiritual and cultural beliefs and practices. Being able to answer the following questions about health beliefs and spiritual beliefs, values, attitudes, and practices with honesty, sincerity, and reflection will help the health care professional uncover any hidden biases and become more sensitive to providing culturally competent care to others.

Spiritual Self-Assessment Questions

The following set of questions can be used as guidelines for assessing spirituality in a cultural context (Martsolf, 1997):

- Who are the most important groups of people in my life right now? In the past?
- Do I belong to any religious or spiritual groups?
- What spiritual beliefs do I share with any of these groups?
- Have I pondered the meaning of life, my relationships with others, the things I value most, my life history, and my future?
- Have I shared any of these thoughts or beliefs with important individuals in my life?
- Do I follow any special rules to express my spiritual beliefs?
- Do I have spiritual rituals that I like to do regularly?

Cultural Self-Assessment Questions

The next questions can be used for assessing cultural beliefs (Engebretson, 1996; Hitchcock et al., 1999; Luckmann, 1999; Lueckenotte, 2000; Martsolf, 1997):

- What are my personal beliefs about people from different cultures?
- What experiences have influenced my values, biases, ideas, and attitudes about people from different cultures?
- Do I associate with culturally diverse people through traveling, reading, attending cultural events, and talking with diverse clients and colleagues?
- What are my health beliefs, values, and attitudes as they relate to health, illness, and health-related practices?
- Do I refrain from making judgments about cultural behaviors and practices that may seem strange to me?
- What are my patterns of communication when interacting with individuals from other cultures?
- Do I respect differences among people of diverse cultures?
- What do I need to do to provide more culturally competent care?

To become more knowledgeable about spirituality, culture, and health, the health care provider must understand the major health belief and health care systems and study the spiritual and health care beliefs of specific cultural groups.

HEALTH BELIEF SYSTEMS

Every culture has it own specific belief system. This belief system provides a framework that influences how individuals view the world, including the cause, prevention, and treatments of illness and the promotion and maintenance of health. Determining which aspects of the belief system arise from an individual's spiritual or religious affiliation and which stem from cultural heritage can sometimes be difficult.

Regardless of whether they originate from spiritual or cultural roots, health belief systems fall into three major categories: scientific or biomedical, magicoreligious, and holistic (Andrews & Boyle, 1995; Dossey et al., 2000; Hitchcock et al., 1999; Leininger & McFarland, 1995; Luckmann, 1999; Miller, 1995).

Scientific or Biomedical Systems

Proponents of a scientific or biomedical health belief system believe that health and illness are controlled by a series of physical and biochemical processes that can be analyzed and manipulated by humans. Four main concepts characterize this type of system:

1. **Determinism:** The view that a cause-and-effect relationship exists for all natural phenomena.
2. **Mechanism:** The view that life is similar to the structure and function of machines, and control can be achieved through mechanical or engineered interventions.
3. **Reductionism:** The view that all life can be divided into isolated smaller parts, such as the division of the mind and the body, to facilitate the study of the whole.
4. **Objective materialism:** The view that only that which can be observed and measured is real.

In the scientific or biomedical health belief system, disease is believed to be caused by physiologic disturbances. Traditional treatment usually involves isolating the faulty "system" and repairing it by placing the individual in a foreign environment (such as a hospital) and administering medication or performing surgery. The health care systems of the United States and many Western industrialized societies are based on this belief system.

Magicoreligious Systems

Followers of magicoreligious health belief systems believe that supernatural forces influence health and illness. They believe the fate of the world depends on God, gods, or supernatural forces. They may view disease or illness as a sign of weakness, a punishment for evildoing, retribution for shameful behavior, a breach of taboo, a loss of the soul, the result of sorcery, or the result of the body's possession by evil spirits. Examples of this type of belief system include the Christian Science religion and some Hispanic, African, and Caribbean healing practices. For example, people from some African-Caribbean cultures believe that parts of a person, such as hair, fingernails, or blood, represent the person and can be used in healing.

Holistic Systems

Those who follow holistic belief systems believe that the forces of nature should be kept in natural balance or harmony. The major premise of these systems is that natural laws govern everything and everyone in the universe. Holistic systems emphasize health rather than the treatment of disease. Wellness and health exist when the person is in harmony with natural laws; illness results from disequilibrium or disharmony.

Chinese medicine and Native American medicine are two examples of holistic health belief systems. Traditional folk care systems are also holistic and depend on home and community resources to help the individual heal or to provide care. Followers of this system go to a hospital only after all else has failed.

HEALTH CARE SYSTEMS

Four health care systems relate to the health belief systems previously described (Dossey et al., 2000; Luckmann, 1999):

1. The **biomedical health care system** combines the Western biomedical health belief system with traditional American values of self-reliance, individualism, and aggressive action. Practitioners receive specialized biomedical training and are legally recognized professionals (such as MDs and RNs).
2. The **popular health care system** involves self-treatment and is the first source of care most people use regardless of their culture. It involves the personal and social networks that determine when to seek care, whom to consult, whether to follow suggested treatments, and how to evaluate the usefulness of such treatments. An individual who goes to a drugstore for over-the-counter flu medication uses this type of health care. Groups such as Alcoholics Anonymous and cancer support groups, while often overlooked by biomedical health care professionals, provide a major source of care for many types of health care problems.
3. The **folk sector or traditional medical system** includes folk healers, such as shamans, curanderos, herbalists, acupressurists, and acupuncturists, as well as healing devices. These healers use a holistic approach to care, are highly trained for their roles, and have a high status in their cultural group. Individuals may use a variety of these health care systems and seek biomedical care only if the other approaches fail or, conversely, initially seek biomedical care and then seek out healers from other health care systems if biomedical treatments fail.
4. The **alternative health care system** includes interventions such as diet therapy (megavitamins and macrobiotics), mind-body control methods (relaxation, hypnotherapy, and prayer), bodywork therapies (chiropractic, massage, and therapeutic touch), and pharmacological and biological therapies (chelation therapy and antioxidants).

CULTURAL GROUPS IN THE UNITED STATES

According to Geiger (2001), health care professionals and spiritual care providers already participate in two cultures:

1. Mainstream society, in which some degree of bias is always a component.
2. The culture of medicine itself, which has its own values, assumptions, and understandings of what should be done and how it should be done.

In addition, health care providers and clients bring their own unique cultural backgrounds to every encounter. For example, many cultures do not have the same understanding of the primarily biological definition of disease dominant in Western medicine. Instead, they may have cultural assumptions about disease and they may believe that informing clients of the potential medical risks of certain procedures needed to treat the disease will influence the outcomes or pose a risk to their health.

Hospitals and health care institutions can be daunting places, even for those individuals who have a health care background. If these individuals are admitted to the hospital, for example, they put their lives into the hands of physicians, nurses, and other allied health care providers. Their daily routines are disrupted. They often experience a sense of helplessness, a lack of control, and fear. For individuals who come from a culture that differs from the traditional Western medical culture or who have poor or insufficient communication skills in English, the experience can be terrifying. In addition, both the client and the health care provider may experience tension as their conflicting belief systems confront one another. Anger, fear, anxiety, or wariness may result.

Nevertheless, the health care staff is responsible for making the individual's experience as comfortable and stress-free as possible by becoming culturally competent. Nursing, social work, and psychiatry are among the many health care disciplines that have joined medical and cultural anthropologists in recognizing the ethnocultural basis of illness and how cultural factors influence health practices (Berger, 1998).

Before health care providers and spiritual care providers can attend to their clients' spiritual needs, they must understand the vast array of cultures and the belief systems that accompany them. Since cultures and cultural issues are so complex and dynamic, health care providers should obtain as much accurate information about specific cultures as possible to enhance their understanding. However, health care providers should guard against the prejudice and stereotyping that result from inadequate information and inattention to context about a culture's beliefs (Bonder et al., 2002).

Although the following sections present each culture as a specific group, it is important to remember that *all members of one culture do not conform to a common pattern; individual characteristics can be found within each cultural grouping.* The information that follows is intended as a broad overview of the major cultural groups. In addition, cultures change over time, so it is important to understand the attributes of a culture at a particular point as well as the historical influences that have affected its development. For example, some people might believe that all African Americans practice voodoo or that all Hispanics use a curandero. Neither statement would be accurate in this day and age. At the same time, "having some basic knowledge about issues that might be important to people of different cultures and religions is useful" (Schott & Henley, 2000, p. 15). For example, health care providers might find it helpful to know that people of a particular faith might observe certain food restrictions.

Because there are so many cultural groups in America and space is limited in one chapter, we have chosen to discuss only a few of the groups with a large population, groups relatively new in their migration status, or groups that hold minority status. In addition to the groups described below, many other cultural groups are represented in the United States.

Blacks/African Americans

The term *blacks* represents a group of highly diverse people who arrived in the United States from all over the world, including:

- The Caribbean
- Haiti

- The Dominican Republic
- Africa

The terms *black* and *African American* are often used interchangeably but this may be incorrect since some people referred to as blacks/African Americans did not come from Africa (Dossey et al., 2000; Luckmann, 1999). While the authors recognize that some readers may wish to differentiate between the two terms, in this chapter the terms will be combined: blacks/African Americans.

Spiritual and Religious Practices

Historically, blacks/African Americans have had to deal with the stress of racial discrimination, poverty, and inner-city violence. However, some have demonstrated a remarkable ability to cope with stress. Research has shown that the negative effects of stress may be offset or counterbalanced by religious involvement. For many blacks/African Americans, religion and religious behavior are integral components of their community (Carter, 2002).

According to Carter (2002), the majority of blacks/African Americans are evangelical Christians with religious experiences originating in the religions of ancient Africa as well as black/African American adaptations of Hebraic, Jewish, Christian (mainly Baptist or Methodist), and Islamic beliefs and rituals. However, many other denominations and religious groups are represented, including Jehovah's Witness, Church of God in Christ, Seventh Day Adventist, Pentecostal, Apostolic, Presbyterian, Lutheran, Roman Catholic, Nation of Islam, and other Islamic sects. These diverse religious beliefs and practices influence the diagnosis and management of both physical and mental disorders.

For many blacks/African Americans, churches and places of worship play a crucial role in survival, and the line is often blurred between the church and the community (Dossey et al., 2000; Koenig, 1999; Musgrave, Allen, & Allen, 2002; Purnell & Paulanka, 1998). Some blacks/African Americans use prayer, laying on of hands, and speaking in tongues in many of their religious practices. Some hold to ancestral beliefs of illness as disharmony with nature and supranormal healing rituals or folk healing (Dossey et al., 2000; Koenig, 1999; Musgrave et al., 2002; Purnell & Paulanka, 1998).

Cultural Issues

The black/African American culture is distinct and encompasses values that may differ from mainstream European American values. Many blacks/African Americans have experienced and struggled against racism and because of a perceived need for solidarity, have sought strength in their family, church, and community (Dossey et al., 2000; Luckmann, 1999). Some have also experienced social injustice, societal inconsistency, and personal impotence, resulting in a profound impact on their character development.

Some core elements of the black/African American character include the following (Dossey, 1997; Purnell & Paulanka, 1998):

- **Self-identity is tied inseparably to that of the group:** The self is considered an extension of the group. The extended kinship group is very important even though individuals are socialized to be in control and independent at an early age.

- **Knowledge includes what is known through the senses and in an extrasensory manner:** For example, rituals, symbols, and language are ways in which knowledge is transmitted from one generation to another.
- **Emotions are expressed naturally and spontaneously in response to experiences:** Blacks/African Americans are highly expressive people as a result of their sense of oneness with life and harmony with nature. Their physical movements are also characterized by a rhythmic sense of balance.
- **Behavior is expressed through subtle patterns of verbal and body language.** Communication may be expressed in "black English" (an informal dialect). However, most black/African Americans are articulate and competent in the formal English language (Dossey, 1997; Purnell & Paulanka, 1998). When communicating, blacks/African Americans may maintain eye contact while speaking to someone but look away while listening to that same individual. Humor is one form of communication found among blacks/African Americans.

The strengths of the black/African American include the following (Leininger & McFarland, 2002; Purnell & Paulanka, 1998):

- A religious or spiritual orientation
- A sense of racial pride
- Resourcefulness
- Family unity, extended family unity, and strong kinship bonds
- A strong work and achievement orientation
- A strong desire for education
- Community involvement

Health Issues and Practices

According to Berger (1998), the collective historical experience of African Americans may explain some of their health preferences and their general distrust of the medical profession. For example, slaves were used as subjects in medical research, the Tuskegee syphilis study subjects were deceived and mistreated, and there was a focus on minority sterilization initiatives in the 1970s. Blacks/African Americans are more likely to believe that hospitals and physicians have a profit motive in deciding treatment choices (Dossey, 1997; Purnell & Paulanka, 1998). Resistance for survival is borne out of generations of adversity (Berger, 1998).

Violence, alcohol and drug use, and weakened family structures have been the result of cultural disruptions. Other health issues for some blacks/African Americans include the following (Leininger & McFarland, 2002; Purnell & Paulanka, 1998):

- The black/African American philosophy of being present oriented, rather than future oriented, is sometimes combined with a fatalistic view about illness and pain.
- Sickle cell disease is the most common genetic disorder among the black/African American population.
- Cancer, cardiovascular diseases, cirrhosis, diabetes, accidents, and infant mortality are the largest contributing factors to the high mortality rates.
- Hypertension is the most serious health problem for blacks/African Americans.

Like many ethnic groups, some blacks/African Americans engage in folk medicine, a traditional method of healing. Extended family members, friends, and neighbors are sought for their advice on illness, caring, and curing (Leininger &

McFarland, 2002). Folk practitioners can be spiritual leaders, grandparents, elders of the community, or voodoo doctors or priests. Some blacks/African Americans believe that "hexes," "sins," "disharmony," and the supernatural can impact their health. Individuals with curative power include the "old lady," "Granny," the "voodoo priest," or the "root doctor." Treatments may include the following (Dossey, 1997; Leininger & McFarland, 2002):

- Teas and cod liver oil
- Herbs and nonprescription drugs
- Oils, incense, candles, and soaps
- Dietary choices
- Laxatives for purging
- Amulets and copper or silver bracelets

Delivering culturally competent care to many black/African Americans means recognizing the following (Witt, Brawer, & Plumb, 2002):

- Coordinating care with "traditional" healers and folk medicine practitioners if appropriate.
- Paying attention to body language and other nonverbal communication.
- Avoiding assumptions about patients and asking about beliefs.
- Providing culturally appropriate health promotion materials.
- Understanding the kinship web and including family members and extended family members in care.
- Avoiding cultural ignorance of the provider.

A Case Study

An African American woman from a southern rural area was wearing a knotted cord around her abdomen when admitted to the hospital for delivery of her child. The delivery nurse said, "You need to remove this string as it is dirty and unnecessary." The nurse removed the cord without the client's consent and started to put it in a garbage container. The client, however, grabbed the cord and put it back on her abdomen saying, "I need this cord to have a safe delivery." After the mother was given anesthesia, the nurse removed the knotted cord and destroyed it. Unfortunately, the infant died during the delivery, and the grieving mother attributed the death of her child to the fact that the nurse "took her cord and killed the child." (Adapted from Leininger & McFarland, 2002, p. 63)

In the preceding case, the staff did not understand why a dirty, knotted cord was so important to their client. Their cultural ignorance and hurtful actions were evident.

Asian Americans

Although this text categorizes all Asian Americans into the same group, each cultural group is very different. Again, this description is intended as an overview and an examination of cultural similarities.

The Asian American culture involves individuals from more than 20 countries who speak more than 100 different languages and represent more than 60 ethnicities

(Dossey et al., 2000). Nearly three-fifths of Asian Americans are foreign-born and originate from the following countries (Luckmann, 1999):

- China
- India
- Japan
- The Philippines
- Korea
- Laos
- Cambodia
- Vietnam
- Thailand
- The Pacific Islands

Spiritual and Religious Practices

Traditional Asian values are based on a wide variety of religious beliefs, including Buddhism, Taoism, Christianity, Confucianism, and Hinduism. These values typically place a higher worth on the interests of the family than on those of the individual. As a result, having a strong group orientation causes some Asian family members to forego their own needs and interests to care for a sick or elderly relative (Dossey et al., 2000; Luckmann, 1999; Purnell & Paulanka, 1998). Education, a strong sense of community, and "keeping up appearances" are also extremely important (Luckmann, 1999).

Cultural Issues

The guiding values of some Asian Americans may include the following (Dossey, 1997; Luckmann, 1999):

- An emphasis on the patrilineal family and the well-being of the community over that of the individual.
- A definition of the family that includes both living and dead relatives related by blood, marriage, and adoption.
- A belief in spirituality and ancestral communication that may involve immortals taking the form of animals or even rocks.
- An emphasis on reciprocity and interdependence but with clearly defined roles and responsibilities for both gender and age; key elements include mutual obligations to others, working and living cooperatively, and group harmony.
- A holistic and multidimensional approach to life and health.
- The concept of "right behavior" (group harmony, support, and well-being), which is connected to maintaining and sustaining friendships, familial bonds, community, and a life lived with interdependence and in perfect order.
- Rituals, such as storytelling, that are powerful therapeutic activities.
- The strategy of seeking a knowledgeable patron or mentor/elder who protects the younger individual from misfortune or erroneous ways.

Health Issues and Practices

According to Berger (1998), Asian health concepts are derived from the central concept of balance between the individual, society, and the universe. The health care practices of some Asian Americans are often profoundly affected by the Buddhist philosophy of life. This philosophy encourages respect for elders and those in authority (such as health care providers), and it teaches that life is a cycle of suffering and rebirth. Because of these beliefs, suffering may be seen as something that must be endured, and some Asian Americans may delay seeking health care remedies. In the Buddhist philosophy, healing is spiritual as well as scientific. Some individuals may believe that their illness is a result of karma as well as biology (Berger, 1998; Purnell & Paulanka, 1998).

Another profound influence on the health of some Asian Americans is the health practice of traditional Chinese medicine. Practiced for more than 3,000 years, Chinese medicine views the mind, body, and spirit as an integrated whole in which each component affects the other. Some Asian Americans believe that the universe is composed of opposing forces: yin and yang, or hot and cold. They believe health is achieved when each element is in balance. In Chinese medicine, herbalists and shamans are considered healers, and they utilize specific foods to maintain harmony with natural forces. They also use techniques that include massage, pinching, and cupping (i.e., the application of cups to the skin to create a vacuum and increase circulation to an area). Cupping may leave physical signs that may be misinterpreted by health care professionals as abuse or injury (Berger, 1998; Purnell & Paulanka, 1998).

Ayurveda (which means "knowledge of life") is another traditional Asian approach to health care. This Indian system of holistic healing views the body as a combination of three forces, or doshas. The basic principle of ayurveda is to prevent illness by maintaining a balance in the body and mind through yoga, meditation, herbal medicine, and dietary recommendations specific for each individual (Shealy, 1996).

Health risk factors for the Asian American can include the following (Dossey et al., 2000; Purnell & Paulanka, 1998).

- The stress of acculturation by Asian immigrants and refugees, especially among the elderly.
- The desire to "keep up appearances," which may delay treatment for mental illness, drug abuse, and domestic violence.
- Lack of knowledge of risk factors or preventive behaviors for diseases such as high blood pressure or cancers .
- Differing expectations of health visits that may deter some Asian Americans from obtaining care (e.g., 90% of the obstetricians and gynecologists in China are female).

When providing culturally competent health care for many Asian Americans, it is important for health care providers to remember the following (Au, 2002; Ngo-Metzger et al., 2003; Philips, 1996):

- The principle of filial piety (i.e., the moral obligation of children to care for and protect elderly parents) is prominent in Asian cultures.
- Chinese medicine teaches that health is a state of spiritual and physical harmony with nature and that a healthy body is in a state of balance.
- The health practitioner can develop trust by establishing and adhering to rules of social conduct and proper social interaction.
- Some Asians use traditional treatment methods or herbal medications and turn to the hospital as a last resort.
- Health care providers should respect the family hierarchy (e.g., addressing the oldest male in a family or group first, before greeting other members, may be appropriate).

- When assessing some Asian families, providers need to gather information regarding specific families' ethnic backgrounds, languages, immigration and refugee experiences, acculturation levels, and community support systems
- Approaching health care from a holistic perspective may be more effective than the traditional Western approach
- When working with some Asian American clients, observing nonverbal cues (such as body language) can often provide important information
- Because some Asians prefer to keep problems within the family, maintaining confidentiality is critical

A Case Study

A Chinese immigrant who had had major surgery was instructed by the nursing staff to "force fluids." The client refused to drink from the pitcher of water that was placed on his bedside stand. The nursing staff threatened the man with intravenous fluids if he didn't take more fluids orally and concluded that the client was uncooperative and noncompliant. When the client's daughter came to visit her father, she told the nursing staff that he would drink hot herbal tea but not cold water. This was culturally acceptable based on the Chinese belief in the use of hot and cold foods and beverages in healing. (Adapted from Habel, 2001)

An understanding of the client's cultural beliefs could have helped health care providers avoid the conflict and confusion.

Hispanic Americans

Hispanic is a broad term that refers to groups with cultural and national identities arising from the following:
- The Caribbean
- Mexico
- Puerto Rico
- Central and South America

Some Hispanic people prefer to be identified by descriptors that are specific to their cultural heritage, such as Mexican, Mexican American, Latin American, Spanish American, Chicano, or Latino (Purnell & Paulanka, 1998). For the purposes of this text, however, the term *Hispanic* will be used.

Spiritual and Religious Practices

Many Hispanics traditionally value religion and believe in self-sacrifice, giving rather than taking, and the acceptance of fate. The predominant religions are Catholicism and Pentecostalism (Dossey et al., 2000). However, some Hispanics are Mormon, Jehovah's Witness, Seventh Day Adventist, Presbyterian, and Baptist.

Religion has a major influence on the health beliefs and practices of most Hispanics. Some Hispanics enjoy talking about their soul or spirit, especially in times of illness. Therefore, it is important for health care providers to be comfortable in communicating and being sensitive to the Hispanic's spiritual beliefs (Dossey et al., 2000; Luckmann, 1999; Purnell & Paulanka, 1998).

Cultural Issues

Despite the variability among subgroups, the Hispanic population in the United States shares some common cultural themes (Leininger & McFarland, 2002; Musgrave et al., 2002):

- Because modern medicine is often viewed as inadequate, some Hispanics commonly visit traditional healers.
- Some Hispanics attribute illness recovery and physician skill to God's power.
- Some Hispanics view health and disease or illness as holistic, including the spiritual, physiological, psychological, social, and metaphysical dimensions.
- Hispanics greatly value the family, and often place the needs of the family above individual needs. Some Hispanics have large extended families with close interpersonal relationships. Family members usually provide abundant physical and emotional support when another family member is ill. During hospitalizations, Hispanics usually want extended family members present, and family members are often involved in decisions about their loved one's care.
- Sometimes older women called *curanderos* serve as health practitioners or provide information about health. Curanderismo is closely enmeshed with religious practice.
- Air, water, foods, herbs, and medicines are believed to have hot-cold properties, but among the Hispanic cultures, there is no uniform consensus as to which substances are hot and which are cold.

The Hispanic culture has certain unwritten rules that govern social interactions. These serve as strengths and protective factors for Hispanic clients, their families, and their communities and include the following (Dossey et al., 2000; Purnell & Paulanka, 1998):

- **La familia** (the family), including parents, siblings, grandparents, aunts, uncles, cousins, compadres, close friends, and godparents
- **Respeto** (respect) and deferential behavior toward others based on age, sex, social position, economic status, and authority
- **Personalismo** (the importance of personal relationships and community)
- **Confianza** (trust)
- **Espiritu** (spirit), mind, and body

Health Issues and Practices

Specific health care issues that may affect the Hispanic client include the following (Leininger & McFarland, 2002; Purnell & Paulanka, 1998):

- A stigma toward mental health in which this disorder is viewed as a sign of weakness (Hispanics have a high incidence of mental health problems, especially depression, anxiety, and substance abuse; contributing factors include the stress caused by immigration, acculturation, and biculturalism [Leininger & McFarland, 2002; Purnell & Paulanka, 1998]).
- Stressors related to social adjustment (including acculturative stress, socioeconomic stress due to inadequate financial resources and limited class standing, and minority stress as a result of racism).
- Environmental health problems from high-risk exposure to ambient air pollution, worker exposure to chemicals in industry, indoor pollution, and pollutants in drinking water.

- Alcohol and substance abuse (especially high in Mexicans and Puerto Ricans) (Leininger & McFarland, 2002; Purnell & Paulanka, 1998).

When providing culturally competent care to Hispanic Americans, it is important to consider the following (Diaz, 2002; Dossey et al., 2000):

- Show respect for clients without being condescending. Respeto is the reciprocal respect between provider and client.
- Be sensitive to the fact that some Hispanic clients are not accustomed to questioning providers.
- Be aware that some Hispanics believe illness may be a punishment for sins or the result of witchcraft, or the evil eye.
- Involve family members, since they are likely to be involved in the treatment and decision-making process for a client.
- Address elders in traditional ways (such as looking below eye level if the patient is older than you are).
- Do not give the impression of being too familiar.
- Nonverbal communication (e.g., a smile or touch) is as important to the client as what may be said.
- Be aware that some members of the Hispanic culture are present oriented and as such, they may neglect preventive health care and may show up late or not at all for appointments.
- Encourage questions, since some Hispanic patients will avoid disagreeing with or expressing doubts with health care providers out of respect.
- Respect traditional healing practices, including the use of spiritual elements such as the worship of saints or the use of talismans.

A Case Study

A Hispanic woman was being treated for tuberculosis. A public health nurse contacted the client by telephone after she missed an appointment. The client informed her she missed the appointment and would not be returning soon because she was seeing a folk practitioner, or curandero, to help cure her disease. (Adapted from Habel, 2001)

Understanding clients' differing health beliefs, such as the use of a holistic holy leader or curandero, is essential in providing culturally competent care.

Native Americans

The term *Native American* implies a uniform culture and healing system. This is not correct.

> The indigenous people of North America identify themselves by nation (commonly called tribe, band or community, clan, and family). The term Native American became a political necessity—a way for similarly oppressed people to identify their unity in a fight for common rights in the face of the encroachment of white military, religious, and educational imperialism. (Cohen, 1998, p. 45)

The Native American (also called American Indian/Alaskan Native) population is growing rapidly, is young, and is geographically scattered. This diverse population includes approximately 530 tribal groups and a wide variety of languages, beliefs, customs, health practices, and rituals. Tribes or clans are the primary social unit and may or may not be blood related. They are a strong source of identity and support (Dossey et al., 2000).

Spiritual and Religious Practices

Native American culture, politics, history, and society are enmeshed with religion. Prior to the continent's occupation by settlers from other countries, Native American tribes each practiced their own unique form of religion. Much of this religious practice has been lost and some Native Americans have assimilated into Western religions. However, some Native Americans still practice folk healing, seeking out the medicine man before going to a health care clinic (Dossey et al., 2000; Purnell & Paulanka, 1998; Taylor, 2002).

Traditional Native American healing systems are holistic ones that focus on balancing the mind, body, and spirit within the context of the community. These healing systems have been practiced for thousands of years and involve a deep sense of connection with place and land. Traditional healing practices also focus on benefits to the emotional, spiritual, psychological, and cultural aspects of the tribe. Often, large communal ceremonies serve to promote the well-being of the entire tribe as the tribal healer reaffirms the group's cultural values. The ceremony involves communicating with the spirit of a disease through prayer and ritual (Cohen, 1998).

Cultural Issues

Native American tribes have survived despite repeated governmental policies of extermination and genocide. These tribes have strong networks, with a deep sense of tribal purpose. They respect and share all ways of healing for all sorts of ills. The strengths and protective factors in Native American families and communities include the following (Cohen, 1998; Dossey, 1997; Struthers & LittleJohn, 1999):

- A strong identification with their culture and heritage.
- A central role of the family in the development of children.
- A deep connection with the past through native stories, group learning, ceremonies, and traditions.
- The use of traditional ceremonies (such as sweat lodge ceremonies, vision quests, talking circles, and spirit camps) that contribute to the healing of the individual, reaffirm community norms, and continue the training and practices of traditional healing.
- Adaptability, strength, and the wisdom to survive.
- Wisdom of and respect for elders.
- Core values of harmony, sharing, hospitality, and giving thanks.
- A belief that illness is due to a lack of harmony, evil spirits, fear and jealousy of other nations, or failure to live according to the code of life.

Health Issues and Practices

Native American healing, spirituality, and culture are intertwined. Spiritual awareness and intuition are a healer's most essential diagnostic tools. Therapeutic healing methods include prayer, music, ritual purification, herbalism, massage, ceremony, and personal innovations of individual healers. Family, friends, and helpers often participate in the healing intervention and help to alleviate the alienation caused by disease (Cohen, 1998).

Providing culturally competent care for Native Americans involves consideration of the following issues (Berger, 1998; Bonder et al., 2002; Cohen, 1998; Purnell & Paulanka, 1998):

- Recognizing the differences between the traditional worldview and the Native American concepts of personal insight, individual awareness, and self-actualization.
- Understanding the profound importance of family and community in healing and illness prevention.
- Understanding the communal effect of traumatic experiences (such as formal boarding schools, imposed religions, economic oppression, or other community events such as an accident, suicide, or death of an elder).
- Understanding and respecting tribal practices and health belief systems; methods of treatment may include prayer, chanting, music, smudging (a cleansing ceremony that involves brushing smoke from herbs or incense over an individual, object, or place), herbalism, laying on of hands, counseling, and ceremonies.
- Understanding that, for some Native Americans, direct eye contact may be considered rude or confrontational, and touch may be considered unacceptable unless the individuals know each other very well.
- Recognizing that there are differences in time perception among the Native American and European American cultures.
- Respecting the practice of speaking in a quiet tone of voice (talking loudly is considered rude).
- Incorporating traditional healing practices into care.
- Listening to community members and adjusting one's thinking and approaches based on their input.
- Becoming part of the circle of healing and fostering relationships with the rest of the healers in the circle.
- Respecting the village, since it identifies the person.
- Waiting and being patient, since the village and its members move at a pace that recognizes the physical and demographic realities of its members.
- Empowering clients so they become self-reliant.

A Case Study

A Navajo mother gave birth to a baby girl in a large urban hospital. When the mother was discharged, she asked for the placenta and umbilical cord. When she learned that they had been destroyed after delivery, she became upset. She had assumed the staff understood the significance of the placenta and umbilical cord and why she needed to dispose of them according to tradition. The mother and her family left the hospital in great distress. (Adapted from Leininger & McFarland, 2002, p. 64)

If the health care professionals had been aware of the cultural importance of the placenta and the umbilical cord, the distress the mother and her family suffered could have been avoided.

Arab Americans

The ancestry of Arabs is traced to the nomadic desert tribes of the Arabian peninsula. Arabic is their common language, and the majority of Arabs practice the religion of Islam. However, Arab Americans are often characterized by diversity of thought, attitude, and behavior, depending on their country of origin. Defined as immigrants from the Arabic-speaking world, Arab Americans come from the following:

- The northern African countries of Morocco, Algeria, Tunisia, Libya, Sudan, and Egypt.
- The western Asian countries of Lebanon, occupied Palestine, Syria, Jordan, Iraq, Kuwait, Bahrain, Qatar, United Arab Emirates, Saudi Arabia, Oman, and Yemen (Leininger & McFarland, 2002; Purnell & Paulanka, 1998).

Spiritual and Religious Practices

Most post-1965 Arab American immigrants are Muslims, practitioners of Islam, the world's largest religion. There are also Christian Arab Americans. Because of Islam's origin in Judaism and Christianity, Christians and Muslims share certain beliefs. However, in Islam, religious faith means "submission to Allah." Worshiping Allah and preparing for the afterlife by fulfilling religious duties as described in the Koran (the Muslim holy book, believed by Muslims to contain God's final revelations to mankind) and the hadith (the oral tradition of the prophet Muhammad; a collection of words and deeds that form the basis of Muslim law) are important practices (Leininger & McFarland, 2002; Purnell & Paulanka, 1998).

Muslims follow the Five Pillars of Islam, which include the profession of faith, prayer, almsgiving, fasting, and pilgrimage (see Chapter 4 for further details on the Five Pillars).

Cultural Issues

The guiding cultural values of some Arab Americans may include the following:

- Privacy is valued and there is resistance to disclose personal information to strangers.
- Families rely more on unspoken expectation and nonverbal cues than overt verbal exchange.
- Individuals believe in predestination and that the events of their lives have been pre-recorded.
- Families are characterized by a strong patriarchal tradition and a hierarchical structure.

Health Issues and Practices

According to research, most conditions that affect the health of Arab Americans are similar to those of the U.S. population as a whole (Purnell & Paulanka, 1998).

The teachings of Islam stress an activist approach to maintaining health as well as an acceptance of God's will. Arab Americans associate good health with eating properly, consuming nutritious foods, and fasting to cure disease (Purnell & Paulanka, 1998).

Many Arab Americans attribute the cause of disease to a multitude of factors, including poor diet, hot and cold shifts, exposure of one's stomach during sleep, emotional or spiritual distress, and envy (the evil eye). The cultural emphasis on modesty may cause embarrassment or an uncomfortable feeling for women who are asked to disrobe for an examination. In addition, some families object to a female being examined by a male physician (Purnell & Paulanka, 1998).

Providing culturally competent care for Arab Americans may include the following suggestions (Leininger & McFarland, 2002; Ott, Al-Khadhuri, & Al-Junaibi, 2003):

- Assess the client's perceptions of his or her health-illness state, taking into account his or her cultural values, beliefs, and patterned life ways.
- Understand that health is very important to some Muslims and the practice of moderation in everything (eating, exercising, working, and praying) is essential to their faith.
- Understand that large numbers of visitors show up at visiting hours and that accommodating this practice is essential.
- Be aware that cultural background, education, and degree of acculturation influence variations in cultural health practice.
- Interpret family members' communication patterns within a cultural context. A family spokesperson may answer questions that are directed toward the client.
- Be aware of Ramadan, the ninth month of the Islamic year, during which Muslims are required to fast from dawn to sunset.
- Be aware that, generally, both male and female Arab patients and their children prefer to be seen by male physicians. However, for pregnancy or gynecological needs, women prefer a female physician.

Two Case Studies

An Arab Muslim man who had recently arrived in the United States was dying. When the nurse entered the man's room, she found several male family members around his bed. The visitors refused to leave the room so she could care for the client. Despite the nurse's objections, they moved his bed so it faced an east window and began praying loudly. The nurse felt she could not give effective care to the client under these circumstances and felt frustrated and ineffective. (Adapted from Leininger & McFarland, 1995, p. 546)

An Arab Muslim mother was told by the nurse in a large children's hospital that she could not remain with her child at night. The Arab mother's response clashed with the nurse when she said, "I must stay with my child while in the hospital." The nurse refused the mother's stay, so the Arab Muslim mother took her child home and did not return. (Adapted from Leininger & McFarland, 2002, p. 58)

In both of these examples, if the nurses had understood the importance of the Arab Americans' beliefs, the outcomes would have been entirely different.

LANGUAGE AND CULTURALLY COMPETENT CARE

The United States is a country of many races and cultures. Providing care to clients with diverse linguistic and cultural backgrounds can be a challenge. The ability to effectively assess the cultural and spiritual beliefs and practices of an individual is based, to a large extent, on the ability to effectively communicate with that individual. Language is the way human beings communicate with each other and is the medium through which spiritual and cultural knowledge about another is obtained. Oral language is a part of every society.

Language and culture are closely intertwined. When working with clients in the health care setting, health care providers may encounter many different languages. Consider the following (Bonder et al., 2002; Luckmann, 1999):

- Language can be problematic in the use of standardized instruments because of vocabulary limitations if the client's first language is not English.
- Language barriers can create communication problems when the provider and the client speak different languages and bring their personal beliefs, values, and cultural backgrounds to the interaction.
- Learning a new language is difficult. Even after years of proficiency, effective use of medical terminology and an understanding of medical concepts may be deficient.
- In times of emotional or physical stress, most individuals for whom English is a second language will revert to their native language.

Whenever a health care provider is involved in an exchange with an individual from another culture, the following dimensions should be considered (Luckmann, 1999):

- How and when to start a conversation
- How best to be understood
- How to respond to the client's gestures or questions
- How to be sensitive to the client's reactions
- How to listen to the client's concerns
- How to take the client's illness and health-related beliefs into consideration in the plan of care

While oral language is one of the most common ways that people communicate with each other, body language or nonverbal communication is an equally important method of communication. Cultural differences and similarities in body language should be considered when communicating with clients from other cultures. For example, many Arabs use nonverbal communication that is contained in the context of the situation, rather than in the verbal words spoken (Dossey et al., 2000; Leininger & McFarland, 2002; Luckmann, 1999).

SUMMARY

Spirituality, culture, and health are inextricably intertwined. They are essential components of every individual, and each one influences the other. Health care professionals cannot address them as separate entities.

Health care professionals and spiritual care providers face many challenges in becoming prepared to administer holistic, respectful, culturally, and spiritually competent care for their patients and clients. They should be aware of and accept cultural differences, have self-awareness, and have understanding and knowledge of a client's culture.

Recognition of cultural diversity is important at all levels of health care and for all practitioners, regardless of where they practice. Equally important, however, is the knowledge that all human beings share certain similarities and an interconnectedness. In a speech given at Arizona State University, His Holiness the Dalai Lama stated,

I think that this is the first time I am meeting most of you. But to me, whether it is an old friend or a new friend, there's not much difference anyway, because I always believe we are the same; we are all human beings. Of course, there may be differences in cultural background or way of life, there may be differences in our faith, or we may be of a different color, but we are human beings, consisting of the human body and the human mind. Our physical structure is the same, and our mind and our emotional nature are also the same. (His Holiness the Dalai Lama & Cutler, 1998, p. 2)

KEY CONCEPTS

1. Current research is beginning to define the complex connections between culture, religious and spiritual beliefs and practices, and an individual's physical and psychological health.
2. Every culture has its own specific belief system. This belief system provides a framework that influences how individuals view the world, including the cause, prevention, and treatment of illness and the promotion and maintenance of health.
3. The diversity of cultures and spiritual expressions in American society requires health care professionals to understand their clients' spiritual and cultural practices in order to provide culturally competent care that effectively addresses their special concerns and health issues.
4. The health care provider's own spiritual and cultural perspectives affect and are affected by all elements of culture; their influence on health and illness cannot be ignored.
5. The ability to effectively assess an individual's cultural and spiritual beliefs and practices is based, to a large extent, on effective communication. Similarities and differences in verbal as well as nonverbal language should be considered when communicating with clients from other cultures.

QUESTIONS FOR REFLECTION

1. Being aware of your own cultural and spiritual values is the first step toward better understanding your clients. Upon completing the self-assessment presented in this chapter on p. 79, did you uncover any hidden biases that might interfere with your ability to provide spiritually competent care? If so, what are one or two steps you could take to dissolve them? (If you did not take the time to complete the spiritual and cultural self-assessment presented in this chapter, please go back and do so now.)
2. In your work or daily activities, you may come into contact with members of a culture or cultures not described in this chapter. If so, what steps could you take to become more sensitive to and learn more about their beliefs, values, and background and provide them with culturally competent care?

References

Alvord, L. A., & Van Pelt, E. C. (1999). *The scalpel and the silver bear: The first Navajo woman surgeon combines Western medicine and traditional healing.* New York: Bantam.

Andrews, M. M., & Boyle, J. S. (1995). *Transcultural concepts in nursing care* (2nd ed.). Philadelphia: University of Pennsylvania Press.

Au, C. (2002). Cultural factors in preventive care: Asian-Americans. *Primary Care: Clinics in Office Practice, 29*(3), viii, 495-502.

Berger, J. T. (1998). Culture and ethnicity in clinical care. *Archives of Internal Medicine, 158,* 2085-2090.

Bonder, B., Martin, L., & Miracle, A. (2002). *Culture in clinical care.* Thorofare, NJ: SLACK Incorporated.

Burkhardt, M. A., & Nagai-Jacobson, M. G. (2002). *Spirituality: Living our connectedness.* New York: Delmar Thomson Learning.

Carter, J. H. (2002). Religion/spirituality in African-American culture: An essential aspect of psychiatric care. *Journal of the National Medical Association, 94*(5), 371-375.

Cohen, K. (1998). Native American medicine. *Alternative Therapies in Health and Medicine, 4*(6), 45-47.

Davidhizar, R., Bechtel, G. A., & Juratovac, A. L. (2000). Responding to the cultural and spiritual needs of clients. *Journal of Practical Nursing, 50*(4), 20-23.

Diaz, V. A. (2002). Cultural factors in preventive care: Latinos. *Primary Care: Clinics in Office Practice, 29*(3), viii, 503-517.

Dossey, B. M. (1997). *Core curriculum for holistic nursing.* Gaithersburg, MD: Aspen.

Dossey, B. M., Keegan, L., & Guzzetta, C. E. (2000). *Holistic nursing: A handbook for practice* (3rd ed.). Gaithersburg, MD: Aspen.

Engebretson, J. (1996). Considerations in diagnosing the spiritual domain. *Nursing Diagnosis, 7*(3), 100.

Geiger, H. J. (2001). Racial stereotyping and medicine: The need for cultural competence. *Canadian Medical Association Journal, 164*(12), 1699.

Habel, M. (2001). Caring for people of many cultures: The challenge for nursing. *NurseWeek.* Retrieved November 20, 2002, from http://www.nurseweek.com/cccc210a.html.

His Holiness the Dalai Lama, & Cutler, H. C. (1998). *The art of happiness.* New York: Riverhead Books.

Hitchcock, J. E., Schubert, P. E., & Thomas, S. A. (1999). *Community health nursing.* New York: Delmar Thomson Learning.

Koenig, H. G. (1999). *The healing power of faith: Science explores medicine's last great frontier.* New York: Simon & Schuster.

Leininger, M., & McFarland, M. R. (1995). *Transcultural nursing: Concepts, theories, research, and practice* (2nd ed.). New York: McGraw-Hill.

Leininger, M., & McFarland, M. R. (2002). *Transcultural nursing: Concepts, theories, research, and practice* (3rd ed.). New York: McGraw-Hill.

Luckmann, J. (1999). *Transcultural communication in nursing.* Albany, NY: Delmar Thomson Learning.

Lueckenotte, A. G. (Ed.). (1996). *Gerontologic nursing.* St. Louis, MO: Mosby-Year Book.

Lueckenotte, A. G. (Ed.). (2000). *Gerontologic nursing* (2nd ed.). St. Louis, MO: Mosby-Year Book.

Macrae, J. A. (2001). *Nursing as a spiritual practice: A contemporary application of Florence Nightingale's views.* New York: Springer.

Martsolf, D. (1997). Cultural aspects of spirituality in cancer care. *Seminars in Oncology Nursing, 13*(4), 231-236.

Matthews, D. A. (1999). *The faith factor: Proof of the healing power of prayer.* New York: Penguin Books.

Miller, M. A. (1995). Culture, spirituality, and women's health. *JOGNN Clinical Issues, 24*(3), 257-263.

Musgrave, C. F., Allen, C. E., & Allen, G. (2002). Spirituality and health for women of color. *American Journal of Public Health, 92*(4), 557-560.

Ngo-Metzger, Q., McCarthy, E. P., Burns, R. B., Davis, R. B., Li, F. P., & Phillips, R. S. (2003). Older Asian Americans and Pacific Islanders dying of cancer use hospice less frequently than older white Americans. *American Journal of Medicine, 15*(1), 47-53.

Ott, B., Al-Khadhuri, J., & Al-Junaibi, S. (2003). Preventing ethical dilemmas: Understanding Islamic health care practices. *Pediatric Nursing, 29*(3), 227-230.

Philips, W. (1996). Culturally competent practice: Understanding Asian family values. Roundtable: Journal of the National Resource Center for Special Needs Adoption, Spaulding for Children, 10(1), 1-2. Retrieved July 24, 2003, from http://www.casanet.org/library/culture/asian-values.htm

Purnell, L. D., & Paulanka, B. J. (1998). *Transcultural health care: A culturally competent approach.* Philadelphia: F. A. Davis.

Schott, J., & Henley, A. (2000). Culture, religion, and patient care. *Nursing Management, 7*(1), 13-16.

Shealy, C. N. (Ed.). (1996). *Physical therapies. The complete family guide to alternative medicine.* Rockport, MA: Element Books.

Struthers, R., & LittleJohn, S. (1999). The essence of Native American nursing. *Journal of Transcultural Nursing, 10*(2), 131-135.

Taylor, E. J. (2002). *Spiritual care.* Upper Saddle River, NJ: Prentice Hall.

Witt, D., Brawer, R., & Plumb, J. (2002). Cultural factors in preventive care: African-Americans. *Primary Care: Clinics in Office Practice, 29*(3), 487-493.

PART II

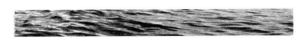

PROVIDING SPIRITUAL CARE

Part II examines the specific tools available to the health care professional in providing compassionate, effective spiritual care. Specifically, this section discusses the various aspects of spiritual care, including:

- Conducting a spiritual assessment and planning, providing, and evaluating spiritual care
- Spiritual therapeutic interventions
- Healing environments

6

SPIRITUAL ASSESSMENT AND SPIRITUAL CARE

"The most spiritual human beings, assuming they are the most courageous, also experience by far the most painful tragedies: but it is precisely for this reason that they honor life, because it brings against them its most formidable weapons."
—Friedrich Nietzsche

LEARNING OBJECTIVES

Upon completing this chapter, you will be able to do the following:
1. Define spiritual care.
2. Describe the components of a spiritual assessment and describe why a spiritual assessment is an important part of client care.
3. Describe strategies that can help ensure a successful spiritual assessment.
4. Discuss several spiritual assessment models.
5. Identify and describe types of alterations in spiritual integrity (spiritual diagnoses).
6. Describe considerations for the planning, implementation, and evaluation of spiritual care.

INTRODUCTION

As the United States becomes more diverse, health care providers increasingly encounter religious and cultural diversity while planning and providing care (Davidhizar, Bechtel, & Juratovac, 2000). With the move toward a more holistic form of care and a rejection—on at least some level—of today's technology-driven health care environment, spirituality now occupies a prominent place in the vocabulary of contemporary health care providers.

Currently, there is a widespread belief that health care providers, especially nurses, should be competent in assessing their clients' spiritual needs, but in reality this is not the case. While many health care providers have been trained to assess and care for the physical, psychological, emotional, social, and cultural aspects of a client, many have not been adequately trained to deal with the spiritual aspect of care. Many professionals feel uncomfortable assessing a client's spiritual beliefs, while others believe that developing an instrument to assess a client's spiritual needs is difficult because of the metaphysical nature of the elements of spirituality (Brush & Daly, 2000; Draper & McSherry, 2002). No universal agreement exists about the definition of spirituality, and the concept can differ among both clients and health care providers (Brush & Daly, 2000; Govier, 2000). This can make spiritual care and spiritual assessment difficult.

In an effort to follow the mandates of regulatory and accrediting bodies as well as a desire to honor their own values and provide the best possible care to clients, health care professionals increasingly recognize that clients want a holistic approach to their care. The influence of the New Age movement has also tapped into a deep need for the spiritual, and more and more people—clients and health care professionals alike—sense that life needs a source of purpose and direction. The role of today's health care professional is to "hear the patient into speech, to be a midwife of the spirit" (O'Connor, 2001, p. 38).

While this chapter offers some guidelines for effective assessment, planning, and implementation, it is important to remember that no single approach to spiritual care and spiritual assessment is likely to meet all the needs of all clients. When discussing the process of spiritual assessment, it is important to be respectful of a broad range of world and religious views and to avoid a "one-size-fits-all" perspective (Draper & McSherry, 2002; Miller, 1999).

SPIRITUAL CARE

Spirituality is deeply personal and involves an individual's deepest fears and aspirations. It provides individuals with a worldview and a context in which to view life and its meaning (Miller, 1999). When people experience a spiritual crisis and need spiritual care, they may choose to discuss their concerns only if they have been shown respect and appreciation (Cobb & Robshaw, 1998). Thus, understanding spirituality and its impact on well-being helps health care practitioners provide compassionate and appropriate spiritual care.

Defining Spiritual Care

Spiritual care involves "promoting an individual's personal integrity, interpersonal relationships, and search for meaning" (Berggren-Thomas & Griggs, 1995, p. 7). It involves the ability of the health care provider to recognize and respond to the multiple aspects of spirituality encountered in clients and their families (Anandarajah & Hight, 2001). Wright (2002) states that spirituality also "affirms the value of each and every individual… and acknowledges the place of cultural traditions and personal relationships" (p. 127).

According to Wright (2002),

- Spiritual care is based on empathy and nonjudgmental love.

- It affirms the worth of each person.
- It responds to both religious and nonreligious needs.
- It involves the humanistic desire to "be there" and listen to another.
- It acknowledges the dignity and nobility of life.
- It respects each person up to the point of death.

Govier (2000) defines spiritual care as care comprised of the "five R's":

- **Reason and Reflection:** The individual in extreme or ordinary circumstances searches for the meaning and purpose in life. Clients in extreme circumstances may ask, "Why is this happening to me?," and the health care provider can help them reflect upon the suffering to find meaning in their lives.
- **Religion:** Religion is the means through which spirituality is expressed via a framework of values, practices, and beliefs. For many people, religion provides the answers to essential questions about life and death. It is important to recognize that many people have their own form of religion that may not fall into the traditional models of recognized religions. These forms still require the respect of health care professionals, whether or not that professional agrees with the individual's beliefs.
- **Relationships:** Relationships with others, the self, or God are at the spiritual center of an individual. He or she may express both vertical and horizontal dimensions of spirituality through transcendent relationships with a Higher Being (vertical) or relationships with others, nature, and the self (horizontal). Thus, creative, meaningful work and service to others can be viewed as one type of spiritual expression.
- **Restoration:** This aspect refers to the ability of a person's spirituality to positively influence his or her physical being. For example, when a particular life event results in an imbalance in a person's physical health, spirituality can help restore that balance by helping the individual understand the meaning of that event. Conversely, when that life event is so devastating that the person cannot restore spiritual balance, that individual may suffer spiritual distress.

Spiritual care can be provided by anyone, but an individual with specialized training in theological beliefs and conflicts usually performs specialized spiritual care. An example of this would be a chaplain trained in CPE (Anandarajah & Hight, 2001).

The Spiritual Care Process: A Systematic Approach

A systematic approach to the spiritual care of any client assures appropriate and effective care. Utilizing this approach means that no step will be overlooked and helps assure that clients will receive the highest quality care possible. It also involves clients in their own plan of care and provides them with a sense of control at a time when they may experience little control over what happens to them (Muncy, 1996).

There are four steps to a systematic approach to spiritual care. Most health care providers are familiar with these steps (Govier, 2000):

1. **Assessing** the individual's spiritual status and identifying specific needs.
2. **Planning** mutually agreed-upon goals for action.
3. **Intervening and implementing** the planned actions.
4. **Evaluating** the individual's status after the intervention.

ASSESSING SPIRITUAL STATUS

Whenever the holistic process is applied to a client's health, assessment is the first step taken. *Assessment* is defined as "the process of gathering, analyzing, and synthesizing salient data into a multidimensional formulation that provides the basis for action decisions" (Hodge, 2001, p. 204). Assessment, diagnosis, and appropriate interventions are the characteristics of excellent client care (O'Connor, 2001). The assessment process, in particular, provides a framework with which to identify the spiritual needs of a client. It allows information to be collected in an efficient, organized manner and then communicated to those who need it (Benedict, 2002).

A holistic approach to a client's spiritual assessment is undertaken with the assumption that spiritual needs influence all other areas of an individual; thus, the assessment will examine the physical, psychological, emotional, social, and cultural components as well (Govier, 2000). Without a thorough and careful assessment, effective interventions are compromised. This is true whether the individual's physical, psychological, emotional, social, cultural, or spiritual dimension is assessed (Taylor, 2002).

Although many health care providers agree that it is important to assess a client's spiritual beliefs as part of a comprehensive, holistic assessment, many of those professionals have a difficult time articulating what spirituality is and, therefore, what spiritual needs actually are (Mansen, 1993). For example, a nurse may know that a client is Catholic and may even know what church the client attends, but knowing the client's religious affiliation does not tell the nurse about the client's spiritual beliefs, spiritual needs, or faith. In addition, health care providers should not assume that an individual without a religious affiliation has no spiritual beliefs (Muncy, 1996). Difficulty may also exist because spirituality in health care today is primarily being delivered from a Judeo-Christian perspective. Others, such as agnostics or atheists, may interpret spirituality from a more humanistic, existential perspective.

The concept of spirituality is deeply subjective; this can make the assessment of spirituality difficult (McSherry & Ross, 2002). However, spiritual needs are not the prerogative of only the believer. The assessment process should embrace the needs of those with no particular religious beliefs, or those who question or dismiss the existence of a Higher Being. This can be accomplished through the use of an open-ended questionnaire and the use of active listening (Govier, 2000).

Why Is Spiritual Assessment Important?

Spiritual assessment is important for several reasons:
- They have been widely shown to be predictive of health outcomes (Miller, 1999).
- They provide important information to the members of the health care team about the individual's ability to cope, about the level (if any) of spiritual distress, and about any interventions that would help that person cope with the health care crisis he or she may be facing (Muncy, 1996).
- They can provide a deeper understanding about a person from a holistic perspective.
- They lead to the delivery of care that respects the individual's health care needs and concerns (Burkhardt & Nagai-Jacobson, 2002). For example,

Burkhardt and Nagai-Jacobson (2002) describe a man who was hospitalized at the insistence of his children after being bitten by a poisonous snake during a religious ceremony at a snake-handling church. He had been at home for the previous several days, being "treated" through prayer and trust in God's healing ability. Upon admission to the hospital, he refused antivenin, even though he knew he might die. Even though this may have been difficult for his health care providers to understand, it was essential that they respect this man's choices and right to his autonomy in light of his religious and spiritual perspectives.

Organizational Mandates for Spiritual Assessment

Multiple organizations mandate the assessment of spirituality. For example, JCAHO specifies that a spiritual assessment should be conducted on all patients. It requires health care organizations to define the content and scope of that assessment. It also requires that the qualifications of the individual(s) performing the assessment be clearly identified (JCAHO, 2001).

According to JCAHO, the spiritual assessment should, at a minimum, determine the patient's denomination, beliefs, and spiritual practices (Davidhizar et al., 2000; JCAHO, 2001). It should also do the following (Benedict, 2002):

- Demonstrate respect for the person's values, religion, and philosophy.
- Include how and when pastoral care is requested and when to provide a list of spiritual resources in the community as well as spiritual leaders who are available on call.
- Provide access to services that ensure religious freedom and availability of services to meet the person's spiritual needs.

In addition, numerous other agencies recognize the importance of spiritual care and spiritual assessment:

- **The World Health Organization**, in its definition of palliative care, states that the control of spiritual problems is of the utmost importance (Wright, 2002).
- **The United Kingdom Central Council for Nurses, Midwives, and Health Visitors'** *Code of Professional Conduct* states that a nurse should "take account of the customs, values, and spiritual beliefs of patients/clients" (McSherry & Ross, 2002, p. 480).
- **The American Nurses Association Code of Ethics** specifies that nurses must provide care that promotes an environment in which values, customs, and beliefs of patients are respected (Davidhizar et al., 2000).
- **The International Council of Nurses Code of Ethics for Nurses** states, "in providing care, the nurse promotes an environment in which the human rights, values, customs, and spiritual beliefs of the individual, family, and community are respected" (McSherry & Ross, 2002, p. 481).
- **The American Association of Colleges of Nursing** recommends that nurse education should provide the nurse with the ability to "comprehend the meaning of human spirituality in order to recognize the relationships of beliefs to culture, behavior, health, and healing" (Cobb & Robshaw, 1998, p. 123).
- **The Canadian Council on Health Services Accreditation** requires the health care team to consider a client's physical, mental, spiritual, and emotional beliefs, and to respect a client's cultural and religious practices as appropriate (VandeCreek & Burton, 2001).

- The American Psychological Association (APA) has a "division for psychologists interested in the interface between religion and psychology" (O'Connor, 2001, p. 36).

Interestingly, the *Diagnostic and Statistical Manual of Mental Disorders* (DSM-IV) has a new category entitled "Religious or Spiritual Problem" that is not considered a mental disorder but is included in the section entitled "Other Conditions Which May Be the Focus of Clinical Attention" (O'Connor, 2001).

The Interdisciplinary Team for Spiritual Caregiving

Several types of health care professionals are capable of conducting a spiritual assessment and providing spiritual care. Physicians and nurses have the opportunity to interact with clients on a constant level. However, everyone on the health care team should be involved in assessing the client's spirituality, including social workers, traditional Western spiritual experts (e.g., hospital chaplains, pastoral care teams, religious ministers), spiritual advisers, and experts of a non-Western orientation (e.g., shamans, medicine men, or spiritual guides).

Family members and members of the individual's religious congregation or spiritual community often provide the primary support for the client (Burkhardt & Nagai-Jacobson, 2002). Various health care professionals who have experience dealing with spiritual concerns can provide guidance and support for the staff, the family, and the client.

PREPARING FOR THE SPIRITUAL ASSESSMENT: STRATEGIES FOR SUCCESS

Several fundamental actions should be completed before the spiritual assessment is undertaken. These actions include performing a spiritual self-assessment, caring for the self in a spiritual way, establishing a positive provider-client relationship, appropriately timing the discussion about spirituality, and creating a "sacred space."

Performing a Spiritual Self-Assessment

The health care provider's ability to assess a person's spiritual needs is related to his or her own spiritual or psychological well-being. An awareness of one's own spirit is essential to providing spiritual care to someone else.

Prior to performing a spiritual assessment on a client, it is important that the health care professional have a firm understanding of his or her own spiritual beliefs, values, and biases (Mansen, 1993). This understanding allows the health care professional to remain focused on the client and helps him or her remain nonjudgmental when dealing with the client's specific spiritual concerns. This is especially important when the client's spiritual beliefs differ from those of the health care professional (Anandarajah & Hight, 2001).

Chapter 5 includes a spiritual self-assessment geared toward identifying spiritual issues within a cultural context. Health care professionals can further examine their beliefs about spirituality by asking themselves the following questions (Burkhardt & Nagai-Jacobson, 2002; Govier, 2000):

- What do I believe in?
- What gives my life meaning?
- What makes me smile?
- What is my favorite part of creation?
- If I could be anywhere, where would I be?
- What do I hope for?
- Who do I love and who loves me?
- When do I feel most connected to others?
- What is my understanding of spirituality?
- How do I express my spirituality?
- What relationship do I have with a Higher Being?
- Why is spiritual care important to me?
- What spiritual rituals are meaningful to me?
- What unique personal qualities can help me meet the spiritual needs of my clients?
- What client-care experiences have left me feeling uncomfortable or inadequate in the area of spiritual care?

A commitment to incorporating spirituality as part of holistic care implies that health care professionals have assessed their own abilities as a listener and addressed any barriers they may experience. Discomfort with any particular view or lifestyle does not make them unsuitable to provide spiritual care. An awareness of this discomfort and its causes can help health care professionals move past the discomfort and barriers and increase their self-awareness. This can facilitate personal and spiritual growth and lead to better care of the professional and the client (Burkhardt & Nagai-Jacobson, 2002).

Caring for the Self in a Spiritual Way

Spiritual self-care is a basic requirement for health care professionals who are asked to care for many clients in today's current health care system. This self-care can take many forms, including involvement in religious practices, community service activities, connecting with family and friends, spending time in nature, meditating, participating in a favorite sport, or spending time alone (Anandarajah & Hight, 2001).

Establishing a Positive Provider-Client Relationship

Since spirituality is such an intimate topic, health care professionals often feel uncomfortable asking clients about their spirituality. However, taking the time to talk with clients about how their spirituality affects their health or illness is important in providing effective care. Most individuals agree that spirituality is different from religiousness, and this may be an important point on which to begin the discussion. Before most clients feel comfortable discussing intimate topics like spirituality, they usually want to have a sense of trust and respect for their health care provider. The health care or spiritual care provider who wishes to develop a sense of rapport and trust with a client will also realize that how spiritual assessment questions are phrased can influence the type of responses received (Koenig, 2001; Sumner, 1998; Taylor, 2002).

When a trusting, therapeutic relationship is established between clients and health care providers, clients are much more likely to feel comfortable discussing their intimate spiritual concerns. The health care provider should be careful, however, in using self-disclosure as a way of establishing this positive relationship. Sharing personal experiences can be interpreted as imposing personal beliefs onto a client, or proselytizing, and may hinder communication. In addition, it is important for health care professionals to explain the reasons for their inquiry and discuss with the client what they plan to do with the information obtained (Govier, 2000).

Appropriately Timing the Discussion About Spirituality

The time at which spiritual questions are asked can help determine the success of the spiritual assessment. For example, most questions are asked when a person is admitted to the hospital or service or seen in a clinic for the first time. When determining the appropriate time for a spiritual assessment, the health care professional should take into consideration the client's overall status. If the individual is extremely ill, the spiritual assessment may need to be deferred until a more appropriate time.

The ability to respectfully and tactfully approach clients about their spiritual beliefs is one that requires skillful interpretation of verbal and nonverbal cues. One way to determine the appropriate time to address spiritual issues is by using Maslow's hierarchy of needs, which states that human beings are inclined to address their physical and safety needs before paying attention to mental and spiritual ones. Following Maslow's hierarchy, for example, the health care provider would not try to initiate a conversation about spiritual beliefs while the client was experiencing intense physical pain or discomfort.

Often, a discussion of spiritual beliefs and practices flows naturally during a discussion of advanced directives; a new diagnosis of a severe, chronic, or terminal illness; end-of-life planning; or during the grieving process (Anandarajah & Hight, 2001). A discussion of spirituality might not be appropriate when an individual is in an area where the interaction will be brief or limited, such as in an acute or day ward. However, it may be very appropriate when the individual will be spending long periods of time in a long-stay, continuous care, or rehabilitation area (Govier, 2000).

Intuition plays an important role in the professional's ability to appropriately interact with clients (Govier, 2000). Intuition is that characteristic that is honed through experience and ability and provides the health care professional with the knowledge needed to determine when and how best to provide spiritual care.

Ideally, a spiritual assessment should be an ongoing endeavor that occurs throughout the provider-client relationship. The results of the spiritual assessment may change over time, so clients should be reassessed regularly, especially if and when their condition changes (Benedict, 2002).

Creating a "Sacred Space"

An important element to consider prior to assessing a client's spiritual needs and during the delivery of spiritual care is the creation of a *sacred space*. A sacred place is a place where one feels safe (Wright & Sayre-Adams, 2000). This concept applies to an inner state of being as well as to the external environment.

Any environment can be transformed into a sacred space through the intent of that transformation and through a "shaping" process that can involve prayer, poetry, expressions of love and concern, dance, rituals, the use of sound or music, candles, incense, the use of color, or through sacred or religious objects (e.g., art, crystals, pictures, or elements of nature) (Burkhardt & Nagai-Jacobson, 2002). While "things" are not sacred in and of themselves, they become sacred when special or reverent sentiments, beliefs, or feelings are attached to them. Ultimately, however, "we do not so much create sacred space, as become and be it. Who we are is the sacred" (Wright & Sayre-Adams, 2000, p. 13).

The presence that a health care provider can bring to the encounter with the client is one of the major factors in creating a sacred space. Wright and Sayre-Adams (2000) state that every healing and caring act is a sacred act, yet most health care providers do their work in stressful, bustling environments that are not often conducive to creating a sacred place of healing. One of the most important things a health care provider can do to create a sacred space is to become still, which permits a reconnection with the senses and provides a connection with the divine. Stillness can be achieved through being in a quiet, still awareness rather than doing something to create that stillness.

Conducting the Spiritual Assessment

When conducting the spiritual assessment, utilizing the following strategies will help ensure the best possible experience (Benedict, 2002; McSherry & Cash, 2000; O'Brien, 1999):

- Sit down with the person and plan the time for the assessment.
- Create a sacred space for the assessment to take place.
- Create an environment of trust and dignity in which the person feels safe discussing personal issues.
- Bring positive intent to the encounter.
- Actively listen to the person (focus on what the person has to say with undivided attention).
- Be nonjudgmental about the individual's beliefs and practices.
- Respect the person and his or her religious or spiritual behaviors through honest and sensitive actions and communication patterns.
- Focus on living rather than on illness and/or dying.
- Use positive nonverbal communication (such as a relaxing manner, leaning slightly toward the client, or an open posture where arms and legs are not crossed).

Spiritual or religious questions may need to be modified or phrased in a way that considers cultural and educational backgrounds. Open-ended questions are the most effective, since they can best help the health care provider assess this complex and unique personal dimension. However, closed-ended questions may be appropriate if the health care provider does not have much time or is inexperienced at completing a more thorough assessment. It is important to explain to the client why these questions are being asked and to describe what you will do with the information obtained. Otherwise, the questions may seem irrelevant and unwelcome (Govier, 2000).

The assessment process should consider and embrace the needs of those who do not have any particular religious beliefs as well as those who question or dismiss the existence of a Higher Being altogether. The use of open-ended questions and active listening techniques and the observation of nonverbal cues (especially facial expressions) can provide the health care professional with information about any fear, doubt, depression, or despair (all indications of spiritual distress) that the client may be experiencing.

MODELS FOR SPIRITUAL ASSESSMENT

Numerous guides, instruments, and scales are used to assess spirituality and religious beliefs, practices, and levels of participation. The ones included in this section provide a wide range of tools based on a broad understanding of spirituality. They can be applied to people from a variety of religious and spiritual perspectives. Some of the instruments are based on a literature review from experts in the field and some are based on qualitative research.

The Informal Assessment

An informal spiritual assessment can be accomplished at any time during a client encounter. Clients often use symbolic or metaphoric language when expressing their thoughts about spirituality, so the health care provider should use active, careful listening skills to interpret what the client is actually revealing. The use of open-ended questions as well as pointed questions about spirituality can provide a great deal of information to the listener who is perceptive enough to hear what is being said (Anandarajah & Hight, 2001).

Examples of elements that could be included, but are not required, in an informal spiritual assessment include the client's denomination, beliefs, and important spiritual practices as well as the following (JCAHO, 2001; O'Connor, 2001):

- Does the client use prayer in his or her life?
- How does the client express his or her spirituality?
- What type of spiritual/religious support does the client require?
- How does the client describe his or her philosophy of life?
- What are the client's spiritual goals?
- What does suffering mean to the client?
- Is a belief in God important to the client?
- What are the names of the client's clergy, ministers, chaplains, pastors, rabbis?
- How has the illness affected the client and his or her family?
- How does faith help the client keep going during the health care experience?

The Formal Assessment

A formal spiritual assessment involves asking specific questions during an interview process to determine what role spiritual beliefs and practices play in the client's illness or recovery, what spiritual needs and resources the individual may have, and how these beliefs and practices may affect the client's treatment plan (Anandarajah & Hight, 2001).

Formal assessment tools need to be easy to use, flexible, and take little time to utilize. They should also be nonintrusive and use wording that encourages the individual to participate in the process. A formal spiritual assessment should not interrogate, alienate, or discriminate between various religious groups. Finally, the assessment should be conducted in a nonthreatening, nonjudgmental manner (McSherry & Ross, 2002).

A brief overview of several formal assessment tools is presented below.

Howden's Spirituality Assessment Scale

Howden's Spirituality Assessment Scale is a 28-item instrument "designed to measure spirituality understood as the integrating or unifying dimension of our being" (Burkhardt & Nagai-Jacobson, 2002, p. 328). This scale provides a broad approach to spiritual assessment that is useful when working with diverse clients. It addresses four specific areas (Dossey, Keegan, & Guzzetta, 2000, pp. 107-108):

1. **Purpose and meaning in life:** The process of searching for or discovering events or relationships that provide a sense of worth, hope, or a reason for existence.
2. **Innerness or inner resources:** The process of striving for or discovering wholeness, identity, and a sense of empowerment manifested in feelings of strength in times of crisis, calmness or serenity in dealing with uncertainty in life, guidance in living, being at peace with one's self and the world, and feelings of ability.
3. **Unifying interconnectedness:** The feeling of relatedness or attachment to others, a sense of relationship to all of life, a feeling of harmony with self and others, and a feeling of oneness with the universe or Universal Being.
4. **Transcendence:** The ability to reach or go beyond the limits of usual experience; the capacity, willingness, or experience of rising above or overcoming bodily or psychic conditions, or the capacity for achieving wellness or self-healing.

The FICA Model

The FICA Model of Spiritual Assessment provides information about what or who gives the client a transcendent meaning of life (Girardin, 2000). FICA stands for Faith and beliefs, Importance and influence of faith and beliefs, Community, and Address in care. This model can be used as a guide for conducting a significant assessment within a short period of time. It includes the following useful questions and areas for assessment (Puchalski & Romer, 2000, pp. 129-137):

Faith and Beliefs

- Do you consider yourself spiritual or religious?
- Do you have spiritual beliefs that help you cope with stress?

If the client responds "No," then you might ask,

- What things do you believe in that give meaning to your life (e.g., family, career, or nature)?

Importance and Influence of Faith or Beliefs

- What influence does your faith have in your life?
- Have your beliefs influenced how you care for yourself?
- What role do your beliefs play in regaining your health?

Community
- Are you part of a religious or spiritual community?
- Is this of support to you and how?
- Is there a person or group of persons that are especially important to you?

Address in Care
- How would you like me, your health care provider, to be involved in the spiritual aspects of your care?

JAREL Spiritual Well-Being Scale

The JAREL Spiritual Well-Being Scale is an assessment tool for nurses based on the study of spiritual well-being in older adults (Burkhardt & Nagai-Jacobson, 2002). However, it has broad application to many types of clients.

The 21 statements from the JAREL Spiritual Well-Being Scale are rated according to a scale ranging from "strongly agree" to "strongly disagree." Statements used in the JAREL Spiritual Well-Being Scale include the following (Hungelmann, Kenkel-Rossi, Klassen, & Stollenwerk, 1996, p. 263):

1. Prayer is an important part of my life.
2. I believe I have spiritual well-being.
3. As I grow older, I find myself more tolerant of others' beliefs.
4. I find meaning and purpose in my life.
5. I feel there is a close relationship between my spiritual beliefs and what I do.
6. I believe in an afterlife.
7. When I am sick, I have less spiritual well-being.
8. I believe in a supreme being.
9. I am able to receive and give love to others.
10. I am satisfied with my life.
11. I set goals for myself.
12. God has little meaning in my life.
13. I am satisfied with the way I am using my abilities.
14. Prayer does not help me in making decisions.
15. I am able to appreciate differences in others.
16. I am pretty well put together.
17. I prefer that others make decisions for me.
18. I find it hard to forgive others.
19. I accept my life situations.
20. Belief in a supreme being has no part in my life.
21. I cannot accept change in my life.

Spiritual Assessment Tool

The interactive Spiritual Assessment Tool was developed by Dossey and Guzzetta (Dossey et al., 2000) and is "based on Burkhardt's critical review of the literature and resulting conceptual analysis of spirituality" (Burkhardt & Nagai-Jacobson, 2002, p. 331). It includes open-ended, reflective questions that can assist health care providers in developing a deeper spiritual awareness for themselves and others. Some of the questions are included below as a sample. The full Spiritual Assessment Tool can be found in *Spirituality: Living Our Connectedness* by Burkhardt and Nagai-Jacobson (2002).

Meaning and Purpose

These questions assess the ability to seek meaning and fulfillment in life, manifest hope, and accept ambiguity and uncertainty.

- What gives your life meaning?
- Do you have a sense of purpose in life?
- What is the most important or powerful thing in your life?

Inner Strengths

These questions assess the ability to manifest joy and recognize strengths, choices, goals, and faith.

- What brings you joy and peace in your life?
- What can you do to feel alive and full of spirit?
- What do you believe?

Interconnectedness

These questions assess your sense of self, sense of belonging in the world with others, capacity for finding meaning in worship or religious activities and a connectedness with a divinity or universe, and connection with life or nature.

- How do you feel about yourself right now?
- Who are the significant people in your life?
- Is worship important to you?
- Do you ever feel at some level a connection with the world or universe?

Qualitative Assessment Tools

While the preceding tools focus primarily on quantitative measures of spirituality, they have been criticized because they "leave little room for clients to negotiate a shared understanding of the individual experiences" (Hodge, 2001, p. 204). Qualitative tools, on the other hand, "tend to be holistic, open-ended, individualistic, ideographic, and process oriented" (Hodge, 2001, p. 204).

Qualitative assessment tools can include taking a spiritual history (similar to taking a family history). A spiritual questionnaire that utilizes a sentence-completion format might consider a topic such as, "I think spirituality is . . ." One such tool asks questions about awareness of the holy, providence, faith, grace or gratefulness, repentance, communion, and the individual's sense of vocation (Hodge, 2001).

Framework for Spiritual Assessment

Hodge (2001, p. 208) suggests a framework for a qualitative spiritual assessment that consists of two portions.

In the **initial narrative framework**, clients are asked about the following:

- The religious/spiritual tradition they grew up with
- The personal experiences and practices that stand out during their years at home and impacted their later life
- Their current spiritual religious orientation

The **interpretive anthropological framework** includes questions in the following six areas:

1. Affect: How does their spirituality affect their life today?
2. Behavior: In what ways do they practice their spirituality?
3. Cognition: What are their current beliefs and how do they affect their life?

4. Communion: What is their experience with the Ultimate?
5. Conscience: How does their spirituality determine right and wrong, impact their key values, and help them deal with guilt and sin?
6. Intuition: Have hunches, premonitions, or spiritual insights affected their life?

SPIRITUAL DIAGNOSES: ALTERATIONS IN SPIRITUAL INTEGRITY

After completing an assessment, it is important to formulate a diagnosis for clients with spiritual needs. Nurses, physicians, mental health professionals, and other spiritual care providers may have a variety of diagnostic labels available to them.

Spiritual Distress

One of the most common diagnoses to result from a spiritual assessment is that of *spiritual distress*, which the North American Nursing Diagnosis Association (NANDA) has specifically identified as a diagnosis (Engebretson, 1996; Wright, 1998). Spiritual distress is described as a state in which an individual is experiencing or is at risk of experiencing a disruption in the values or beliefs that provide the individual with strength, hope, and meaning (Berggren-Thomas & Griggs, 1995).

Identified as "any disruption—or disease—in one's spirit" (Taylor, 2002, p. 138), spiritual distress is "the disruption in the life principle that pervades a person's entire being and that transcends one's biological and psychological nature. In other words, it means the person's self is disintegrating" (Benedict, 2002, p. 7). Spiritual distress or a spiritual crisis occurs when people cannot find meaning, hope, love, peace, or strength in their lives. It occurs when a lack of connection to life or people occurs and when their life situation is in conflict with their beliefs (Anandarajah & Hight, 2001).

Clients in spiritual distress may say they are "brokenhearted" or their "spirits are down," may talk about feelings of being abandoned by God or by others, or may have doubts about religious or spiritual beliefs. A client may say, "I don't know why I got this illness. There must be some reason" (Davidhizar et al., 2000).

Specific characteristics of spiritual distress include the following (Benedict, 2002; Taylor, 2002):

- Questions about the moral/ethical implications of a therapeutic regimen
- Feelings of worthlessness, bitterness, denial, guilt, and fear
- Nightmares and/or sleep disturbances
- Anorexia
- Somatic complaints
- Verbalization of inner conflicts about beliefs
- Inability to participate in usual religious practices
- Seeking of spiritual assistance
- Questioning the meaning of suffering
- Questioning the meaning of one's existence
- Anger toward God
- Alterations in mood/behavior (anger, crying, withdrawal, anxiety, apathy, etc.)
- Gallows humor

Spiritual distress or crisis can impact an individual's physical and mental health and is often precipitated by a medical illness or impending death (Anandarajah & Hight, 2001). Additional risk factors for spiritual distress include the following (Taylor, 2002):

- Loss of a loved one
- Low self-esteem
- Mental illness
- Natural disasters
- Physical illnesses
- Situational losses
- Substance abuse
- Poor relationships with others
- Physical or psychological stress
- Inability to forgive (either the self or others)
- Lack of self-love
- Extreme anxiety

When caring for a person in spiritual distress, the health care provider should seek to help the individual participate in care and in activities with others, verbalize a more positive self-concept, realize he or she is not to blame for illness, discuss values and beliefs regarding spiritual issues, and actively seek positive relationships (Burkhardt & Nagai-Jacobson, 2002). This can be achieved by implementing specific interventions such as the following (Burkhardt & Nagai-Jacobson, 2002):

- Determining the spiritual or religious orientation and influence of the client's and family's belief systems.
- Noting expressions of the inability to find meaning in life.
- Listening to expressions of anger or alienation from God.
- Providing a sacred space for the individual to express his or her concerns.
- Expressing acceptance of the client's beliefs.
- Asking how you might be most helpful to the client.
- Developing a therapeutic relationship with the client and the family.
- Helping the client and/or the family find spiritual/religious resources and support.

Additional Diagnoses

While spiritual distress is one of the most common problems of spiritual integrity, other diagnoses specific to the nursing profession related to alterations in spiritual integrity include the following (O'Brien, 1999, pp. 69-70):

- **Spiritual pain:** The expression of discomfort or suffering related to one's experience with God. Spiritual pain can be expressed through feelings of a lack of fulfillment or a lack of peace in terms of the relationship to one's creator. It can be expressed through a statement such as, "I am not living according to God's will."
- **Spiritual alienation:** The feeling that God seems very far away or remote from one's everyday life. The individual often expresses feelings of spiritual alienation and a negative attitude toward receiving any spiritual comfort or help from God. This problem can be expressed through a statement such as, "Where is God when I need him?"

- **Spiritual anxiety:** A fear that God is displeased with the individual's behavior. It is usually exhibited through expressions of fear of God's anger or punishment, such as, "This is God's punishment for my faults."
- **Spiritual guilt:** A fear that the individual has failed to do the things that should be done in a spiritual life.
- **Spiritual anger:** Frustration, anguish, or outrage directed at God for allowing trials, sickness, or perceived unfairness.
- **Spiritual loss:** A feeling of emptiness regarding spiritual matters. It is expressed through psychological depression or feelings of powerlessness or uselessness.
- **Spiritual despair:** A feeling that God no longer cares. It is evidenced by expressing the idea that there is no hope of having a relationship with God.

PLANNING SPIRITUAL CARE

Once the assessment has been completed, the information gained can be used to formulate an effective plan of spiritual care. A spiritual care plan should reflect the needs identified during the assessment phase. The information should be verified with the client, and then realistic, client-centered goals should be set within a time frame that is acceptable to both the client and the health care or spiritual care provider. Many health care providers feel uncomfortable with planning spiritual interventions because of a fear of imposing their own personal beliefs or because of a lack of training or knowledge of the client's beliefs, practices, and rituals of religion (O'Neill, 2002). Effective communication between the client, family, friends, and other members of the health care team is essential (Govier, 2000; McSherry & Cash, 2000).

Spiritual health affects physical and psychological health and, therefore, should be given a high priority when planning care, especially if the client is diagnosed with spiritual distress (Taylor, 2002). Spiritual caregiving can include four areas (Brush & Daly, 2000):

1. **Affirmation:** The acknowledgement of factors in a client's life that could be considered positive.
2. **Therapeutic communication:** "Listening" to the meaning of the client's conversation through astute observation of body language and facial expressions and through maintaining an active "presence" with the client.
3. **Reminiscence:** A life review that allows the client to discuss people, places, or situations that are/were meaningful in his or her life.
4. **Referral:** The appropriate recommendation to a spiritual health care provider, such as clergy.

In planning for spiritual care, several options may be considered by the health care provider (Anandarajah & Hight, 2001; McSherry & Cash, 2000):

- Take no further action except offering one's presence, understanding, compassion, and acceptance of the client. This can mean allowing the client time to pray or read in private, arranging care so the client can attend a communion service, or contacting the client's religious or spiritual leaders for support.
- Incorporate spirituality into preventive health care measures by helping the client identify and utilize his or her spiritual resources. This can mean helping the client work through spiritual issues with a chaplain or spiritual adviser or

providing information about spiritual resources in the city or town in which the client is hospitalized.

- Incorporate spirituality in conjunction with standard health care treatments. This can involve allowing a spiritual adviser or medicine man to conduct specific spiritual rituals for the client.
- Modify the treatment plan as needed once the spiritual needs of the client are understood.

IMPLEMENTING SPIRITUAL CARE

Following a spiritual assessment and the development of a plan of care, the goals or outcomes that have been set can now be implemented. This requires committing energy and time to the goals, which may present a challenge to the health care or spiritual care provider who is unable to spend much time with a client or who is already overwhelmed with the demands of an understaffed or busy hospital ward or community setting. In fact, many spiritual conversations with people in the hospital take place at night when nurses, in particular, have more time and are freed from the daily routine tasks that may prevent them from having this type of discussion during a day shift. In addition, many clients feel more vulnerable and alone during the night and are more willing to discuss these types of issues than during the daytime (Govier, 2000; O'Neill, 2002).

Interventions can include the following actions (Dossey et al., 2000; Taylor, 2002):
- Caring touch
- Fostering connectedness between the client and his or her family, friends, or pets
- Analyzing dreams
- Reading spiritually uplifting materials, including sacred writings
- Utilizing art as a means of expressing spiritual thoughts and beliefs
- Facilitating the use of spiritual rituals
- Utilizing humor
- Utilizing imagery, meditation, or prayer
- Encouraging journal writing or scrapbook making
- Encouraging experiences in nature
- Incorporating storytelling, reminiscing, or life review into care plans

Other effective tools for implementing spiritual care include the use of intuition and appropriate behavioral interventions, both of which depend on the level of self-awareness possessed by the health care professional. Health care professionals should recognize and understand their own limitations and utilize other available professional resources wherever and whenever appropriate (Govier, 2000).

EVALUATING SPIRITUAL CARE

Once all the other steps have been completed, an evaluation of those steps is necessary to determine their effectiveness. Because the spiritual dimension is a subjective one, this step can be somewhat imprecise and difficult. While it is simple to measure the effectiveness of, for example, the administration of antibiotics for an infection, it can be quite difficult to measure cause and effect as they relate to a spiritual intervention. Consultation with the client and participation in the spiritual interventions are two factors that help determine their effectiveness.

Perhaps the most obvious way to measure the effectiveness of spiritual intervention is to ask the client directly, and carefully observe his or her physical, verbal, or nonverbal cues (Govier, 2000; McSherry & Cash, 2000; Taylor, 2002). For example, the health care provider can observe whether a client attends a particular service or document that the client's spiritual/religious leader came to visit.

One difficulty with evaluating whether or not spiritual goals were achieved is the time frame involved in achieving them. It may take an individual many months to resolve a health problem or personal crisis. It is unrealistic to expect a client to reflect, adjust, and regain his or her spiritual balance in a matter of hours, days, or even weeks. Thus, the specific spiritual needs of a client should be carefully considered and time frames for implementation and evaluation of spiritual goals realistically decided (McSherry & Cash, 2000).

If It Wasn't Charted, It Wasn't Done

There is an old adage about documentation: If it wasn't charted, it wasn't done. This applies to spiritual care as well as to every other aspect of care. JCAHO requires documentation of spiritual care, and most hospital admission forms have some areas where spirituality can be assessed and addressed. Documentation about the spiritual care provided serves several purposes (Taylor, 2002):

- It allows health care professionals to communicate with each other about what has been identified as a spiritual need, what interventions were planned, what interventions were effective, and the client's response to the care.
- It supports auditing and quality assurance requirements for health care accreditation.
- It provides researchers and analysts with information that will ultimately improve health care.

SUMMARY

Spirituality is a complex, multidimensional part of the human experience and is difficult to fully understand or measure using traditional scientific methods. However, spirituality is an important part of the overall plan of care for any client. While study is underway to determine its exact effects on health and well-being, responsible health care and spiritual care providers will continue to address this aspect of health through assessment, planning, implementation, and evaluation of care.

KEY CONCEPTS

1. Since no universal agreement exists about what spirituality "means" and the concept can differ among both clients and health care providers, spiritual care and spiritual assessment are difficult. No single approach to spiritual care and spiritual assessment is likely to meet all the needs of all clients.

2. Spiritual care responds to both religious and nonreligious needs and it promotes an individual's personal integrity, interpersonal relationships, and search for meaning.
3. There are four steps to a systematic approach to spiritual care: assessing spiritual needs, planning spiritual goals, intervening and implementing planned actions, and evaluating the individual's status after the interventions.
4. A commitment to incorporating spirituality as part of holistic care implies that health care providers have assessed their own ability as a listener and addressed any barriers that they may experience.
5. Spiritual distress is one of the most common problems of spiritual integrity, although other alterations in spiritual integrity can include spiritual pain, spiritual alienation, spiritual anxiety, spiritual guilt, spiritual anger, spiritual loss, and spiritual despair.
6. As in other areas of care, thorough documentation of the care provided is a necessary part of the spiritual care process.

QUESTIONS FOR REFLECTION

1. To support the "whole" person, health care providers should be willing and able to address their clients' spiritual needs. How do you feel about discussing such matters with your clients?
2. If you feel uncomfortable about addressing the issue of spirituality, is there someone with whom you can discuss these matters and perhaps alleviate your discomfort so you can better serve your clients?

REFERENCES

Anandarajah, G., & Hight, E. (2001). Spirituality and medical practice: Using the HOPE questions as a practical tool for spiritual assessment. *American Family Physician, 63*(1), 81-89.

Benedict, L. M. (2002). *Spiritual assessment: EDA 318-0479.* Carrollton, TX: PRIMEDIA Healthcare: Long Term Care Network.

Berggren-Thomas, P., & Griggs, M. J. (1995). Spirituality in aging: Spiritual need or spiritual journey? *Journal of Gerontological Nursing, 21*(3), 5-10.

Brush, B. L., & Daly, P. R. (2000). Assessing spirituality in primary care practice: Is there time? *Clinical Excellence for Nurse Practitioners, 4*(2), 67-71.

Burkhardt, M. A., & Nagai-Jacobson, M. G. (2002). *Spirituality: Living our connectedness.* Albany, NY: Delmar Thomson Learning.

Cobb, M., & Robshaw, V. (1998). *The spiritual challenge of health care.* Edinburgh: Churchill Livingstone.

Davidhizar, R., Bechtel, G. A., & Juratovac, A. L. (2000). Responding to the cultural and spiritual needs of clients. *Journal of Practical Nursing, 50*(4), 20-23.

Dossey, B. M., Keegan, L., & Guzzetta, C. E. (2000). *Holistic nursing: A handbook for practice.* Gaithersburg, MD: Aspen.

Draper, P., & McSherry, W. (2002). A critical view of spirituality and spiritual assessment. *Journal of Advanced Nursing, 39*(1), 1-2.

Engebretson, J. (1996). Considerations in diagnosing in the spiritual domain. *Nursing Diagnosis, 7*(3), 100-108.

Girardin, D. W. (2000). Integration of complementary disciplines into the oncology clinic, part IV: Implications for spirituality with oncology patients. *Current Problems in Cancer, 24*(5), 268-279.

Govier, I. (2000). Spiritual care in nursing: A systematic approach. *Nursing Standard, 14*(17), 32-36.

Hodge, D. R. (2001). Spiritual assessment: A review of major qualitative methods and a new framework for assessing spirituality. *Social Work, 46*(3), 203-214.

Hungelmann, J., Kenkel-Rossi, E., Klassen, L., & Stollenwerk, R. (1996). Focus on spiritual well-being: Harmonious interconnectedness of mind-body-spirit—Use of the JAREL Spiritual Well-Being Scale. *Geriatric Nursing, 17*(6), 262-266.

Joint Commission on Accreditation of Healthcare Organizations. (2001). Spiritual assessment. Retrieved June 16, 2002, from http://www.jcaho.org/accredited+organizations/behavioral+ health+care/standards/faqs/provision+of+care/assessment/spiritual+assessment+.htm.

Koenig, H. G. (2001). Religion, spirituality, and medicine: How are they related and what does it mean? *Mayo Clinic Proceedings, 76*(12), 1189-1191.

Mansen, T. J. (1993). The spiritual dimension of individuals: Conceptual development. *Nursing Diagnosis, 4*(4), 140-147.

McSherry, W., & Cash, K. (2000). *Making sense of spirituality in nursing practice.* Edinburgh: Churchill Livingstone.

McSherry, W., & Ross, L. (2002). Dilemmas of spiritual assessment: Considerations for nursing practice. *Journal of Advanced Nursing, 38*(5), 479-488.

Miller, W. R. (Ed.). (1999). *Integrating spirituality into treatment.* Washington, DC: American Psychological Association.

Muncy, J. F. (1996). Muncy comprehensive spiritual assessment. *American Journal of Hospice & Palliative Care, 13*(5), 44-45.

O'Brien, M. E. (1999). *Spirituality in nursing: Standing on holy ground.* Boston: Jones & Bartlett.

O'Connor, C. I. (2001). Characteristics of spirituality, assessment, and prayer in holistic nursing. *Nursing Clinics of North America, 36*(1), 33-42.

O'Neill, P. A. (2002). *Caring for the older adult: A health promotion perspective.* Philadelphia: W. B. Saunders.

Puchalski, C. M., & Romer, A. L. (2000). Taking a spiritual history allows clinicians to understand patients more fully. *Journal of Palliative Medicine, 3*, 129-137.

Sumner, C. H. (1998). Recognizing and responding to spiritual distress. *American Journal of Nursing, 98*(1), 26-31.

Taylor, E. J. (2002). *Spiritual care: Nursing theory, research, and practice.* Upper Saddle River, NJ: Prentice Hall.

VandeCreek, L., & Burton, L. (2001). *Professional chaplaincy: Its role and importance in healthcare.* New York: Association for Clinical Pastoral Education, Association of Professional Chaplains, Canadian Association for Pastoral Practice and Education, National Association of Catholic Chaplains, National Association of Jewish Chaplains.

Wright, K. B. (1998). Professional, ethical, and legal implications for spiritual care in nursing. *Image: Journal of Nursing Scholarship, 30*(1), 81-83.

Wright, M. C. (2002). The essence of spiritual care: A phenomenological enquiry. *Palliative Medicine, 16*(2), 125-132.

Wright, S. G., & Sayre-Adams, J. (2000). *Sacred space: Right relationship and spirituality in healthcare.* London: Harcourt Publishers Limited.

7

THERAPEUTIC INTERVENTIONS FOR HEALING

"Music is well said to be the speech of angels: in fact, nothing among the utterances allowed to man is felt to be so divine. It brings us near to the infinite."
—Thomas Carlyle (1795-1881)

LEARNING OBJECTIVES

Upon completing this chapter, you will be able to do the following:
1. Describe the therapeutic uses, beneficial effects, and physiological responses of music.
2. List the types of music therapy intervention.
3. Describe art therapy interventions and settings in which they are utilized.
4. List the goals, types of interventions, and benefits of dance and movement therapy.
5. Describe the psychological, physiological, and spiritual benefits of laughter and therapeutic humor.
6. Differentiate between the types of therapy animals and describe three theories that explain the effects of animal-assisted therapy on health and well-being.

INTRODUCTION

Music, art, dance, humor, and animals all have the ability to soothe, comfort, heal, and lift the spirits. These healing interventions have a powerful effect on an individual's physical, spiritual, and mental health. Most people engage in these activities without being fully aware of the beneficial effects on their health and well-being.

Music has been used to facilitate healing throughout history and has been a vital part of all societies and cultures. For example, Aristotle believed the flute was powerful. Pythagoras taught his students to change their emotions of worry, fear, sorrow, and anger by singing and playing a musical instrument daily. Modern-day music therapy began after World War I when community musicians played for hospitalized veterans. Those who attended the concerts demonstrated a significant change in their physiological and emotional well-being. Today, music is integrated as a spiritual practice in compassionate health care (Updike, 1998).

Art has been used as a visual means of communication and expression since prehistoric times. Art therapy began as a treatment modality in the 1930s when the healing potential of artistic self-expression was realized and integrated into the fields of psychology and art. The use of art therapy can help to clarify an individual's existential/spiritual issues (Gabriel et al., 2001).

Dance is universal. Throughout the world, people have danced to celebrate, to bond together as communities, to share sentiments, and to heal the sick. Dance therapy is concerned with genuine, creative movement and the objective of establishing unity of mind, body, and spirit. Dance is the essence of embodiment (Block & Kissell, 2001).

Humor is a complex phenomenon and an essential part of human relationships. According to anthropologists, no culture that is devoid of humor has ever been found at any time in history. A sense of humor involves not only a perspective on life (a way of perceiving the world), it is also a behavior that expresses that perspective (Wooten, 2000).

Animals have been used in cultures throughout the world for therapeutic purposes for thousands of years, and their use is increasing in hospitals, nursing homes, and psychiatric institutions. AAT is being used more and more often to treat acutely and chronically ill clients (Stanley-Hermanns & Miller, 2002).

This chapter will explore each of these disciplines and their application as therapeutic interventions for healing.

MUSIC THERAPY

Music, which is an integral part of most religious worship services across cultures and denominations, can soothe the spirit; provide a means of focusing on spiritual awareness; and lift an individual to a place of peace, serenity, and inner awareness. In addition, music decreases anxiety, depression, agitation, and aggression and increases relaxation and a positive mood (Cabrera & Lee, 2000; Taylor, 2002).

Music therapy is defined as the behavioral science concerned with the systematic application of music to produce relaxation and desired changes in emotions, behavior, and physiology (Dossey, Keegan, & Guzzetta, 2000). It is an allied health service similar to occupational therapy and physical therapy, and it utilizes music therapeutically to address physical, psychological, cognitive, and/or social functioning. Music therapy complements traditional therapy, encourages active participation in one's own health care, and provides an integrated mind-body experience. As a therapeutic modality, music can be used to engage the spiritual dimension (Updike, 1998).

Music is not only a medium of expression unique to each culture, it is also recognized as a powerful medium that affects human health. Music therapy is recognized as a viable treatment modality by the Health Care Financing Administration (HCFA), JCAHO, the Commission on Accreditation of Rehabilitation Facilities (CARF), and the National Rehabilitation Caucus (NRC).

In 1998, the American Music Therapy Association (AMTA) was founded as a result of the unification of the American Association for Music Therapy (founded in 1971) and the National Association for Music Therapy (founded in 1950). The AMTA establishes criteria for the education and clinical training of music therapists.

In an age in which more and more individuals are turning to holistic methods of healing, music therapy is a powerful and nonthreatening medium. Music therapy is used successfully with individuals of all ages and disabilities. For example, music therapy often complements the treatment provided for individuals with neurological conditions, including brain injury, stroke, and Parkinson's and Alzheimer's diseases. Music therapy can improve the mobility of stroke patients, lift depression and anxiety, and even lessen the amount of anesthesia needed by women during childbirth (Matthews & Clark, 1998).

Principles of Sound

Understanding the principles of sound is essential to appreciating music's capacity to achieve therapeutic psychophysiological and spiritual outcomes. Sound is produced when an object vibrates in a random or periodic repeated motion. Sound is perceived by the human ear and through skin and bone conduction. Other senses, such as sight, smell, and touch, allow individuals to perceive an even wider range of vibrations than by hearing alone (Dossey et al., 2000).

The study of patterns of shapes evoked by sound is called cymatics. According to cymatics, matter assumes certain shapes or patterns based on the vibrations or frequency of the sound to which it is exposed. For example, the form of a snowflake may take on its shape in response to sounds in nature. In a similar way, the human body is a system of vibrating atomic particles acting as a vibratory transformer that gives off and takes in sound from the environment. Music can act as an environmental pacemaker by speeding up or slowing down heart rate, brainwaves, and respirations. The result is a gradual entrainment (or synchronization) of the body's vibrations with those of the music, resulting in a change in an individual's psychophysiological state (Dossey et al., 2000).

According to Updike (1998), "The nature of human physical, emotional, and spiritual patterns can be defined by their activity and interactions" (p. 65). Conceived as vibratory matter, music may serve as a profound and tangible medium for balancing the emotional and physiologic essence of the whole body. Vibration is the essence of sound and is dynamic (Updike, 1998).

Physiological Responses to Music

The type of music played (such as soothing music) may determine the physiological changed produced. Soothing music may alter an individual's perception of time and can produce a hypometabolic response similar to a relaxation response in which autonomic, immune, endocrine, and neuropeptide systems are altered (Achterberg, Dossey, & Kolkmeir, 1994; Dossey et al., 2000).

Music heals but is not prescriptive because its power varies according to the composition, the performer, the listener, the posture assumed in listening, and additional factors. A complete understanding of how music heals would require an examination of what music does and some of its therapeutic effects. Listed below are some of music's possible uses and beneficial effects (Campbell, 2001).

Music Masks Unpleasant Sounds and Feelings

Many dental professionals understand the effects of music; they use it to mask the sound of the drill and dispel the uncomfortable feeling created by the harsh sounds and vibrations of their dental instruments.

Music Can Slow Down and Equalize Brainwaves

Beta waves occur during ordinary consciousness and vibrate from 14 to 20 hertz (Hz). Alpha waves occur during periods of heightened awareness and calm and cycle from 8 to 13 Hz. Theta waves occur during periods of peak creativity, meditation, and sleep and cycle from 4 to 7 Hz. Delta waves occur during deep sleep, deep meditation, and unconsciousness and range from 0.5 to 3 Hz. Listening to certain types of music, such as Baroque, New Age, and other ambient (with no dominant rhythm) music, can shift consciousness from the beta stage toward the alpha range. Shamanic drumming can take the listener into the theta range.

Music Affects Respiration

Breathing at a deep, slow rate is optimal and contributes to calmness. Listening to music with longer, slower sounds can cause an individual's breathing to deepen and slow, creating a calm, relaxed sensation. Gregorian chant, New Age, and ambient music can create this effect.

Music Affects the Heartbeat, Pulse Rate, and Blood Pressure

Musical variables such as frequency, tempo, and volume tend to speed up or slow down heart rate. The faster the music, the faster the heart rate; the slower the music, the slower the heart rate. A slower heartbeat calms the mind, creates less physical tension and stress, and helps the body heal itself. Listening to music with a frequency of 44 to 55 Hz can lower an individual's blood pressure.

Music Reduces Muscle Tension and Improves Body Movement and Coordination

Through the autonomic nervous system, the auditory nerve connects the inner ear with all the muscles in the body. Thus, muscle strength, flexibility, and tone are influenced by sound and vibration. Music is used in recovery wards and rehabilitation clinics to restructure repetitive movements following accidents and illness.

Music Affects Body Temperature

Loud music with a strong beat can raise body temperature by a few degrees; soft music with a weak beat can lower it.

Music Can Increase Endorphin Levels

Endorphins, the proteins that occur naturally in the brain, can lessen pain and induce a "natural high." Music can stimulate the release of endorphins, which can then decrease the need for pain medication, provide distraction from pain, and relieve anxiety.

Music Can Regulate Stress-Related Hormones

Listening to relaxing, ambient music may reduce the level of stress hormones in the blood, which in some cases may reduce or replace the need for medication.

Music and Sound Can Boost Immune Function

Insufficient oxygen in the blood may be a major cause of immune deficiency and degenerative disease. Listening to certain types of music as well as engaging in singing, chanting, and other vocal forms relax muscles and improve respiratory effort, resulting in better oxygenation of the cells.

Therapeutic Uses and Benefits of Music

Music therapy can be used in all types of health care settings, from the birthing to the dying process. Music is used in hospitals for several reasons (Cabrera & Lee, 2000; Campbell, 2001; Dossey et al., 2000):

- To alleviate pain in conjunction with anesthesia or pain medication
- To reduce anxiety during labor and delivery
- To control the sensitive environment of the neonate
- To elevate clients' moods and counteract depression
- To promote movement for physical rehabilitation
- To calm or sedate clients
- To induce soothing, relaxing sensations
- To induce sleep, counteract apprehension or fear, and lessen muscle tension for the purpose of relaxation

In nursing homes, music is used to increase or maintain elderly clients' level of physical, mental, spiritual, and social/emotional functioning and improve their quality of life (Campbell, 2001; Dossey et al., 2000).

Music is used in psychiatric facilities to help clients explore their personal feelings, make positive changes in their mood and emotional states, gain a sense of control over life through successful experiences, practice problem solving, and resolve conflicts leading to stronger family and peer relationships (Campbell, 2001; Dossey et al., 2000).

Using a planned and systematic approach to the use of music and music activities, music therapy interventions for the mind, body, and spirit provide opportunities for the following (Campbell, 2001; Dossey et al., 2000; Schroeder-Sheker, 1994):

- Anxiety and stress reduction
- Nonpharmacological management of pain and discomfort
- Positive changes in mood and emotional states
- Active and positive client participation in treatment
- Enhanced awareness of self and environment
- Development of coping and relaxation skills
- Improved emotional intimacy with families and caregivers
- Meeting the complex physical and spiritual needs of the dying
- Relaxation for the entire family
  Increased or improved meaningful time spent together in a positive, creative way

Music Therapy Interventions

Music therapy is used to address the physical, psychological, spiritual, cognitive, and social needs of individuals with disabilities and illnesses. As Updike (1998) writes, "Music as a spiritual dimension is far more substantive than a mere whimsical statement. Intentional use of music to engage a sacred dimension does not guarantee the experience, but renders it more accessible" (p. 64).

After assessing the needs and personal preferences of each client, a qualified music therapist provides the appropriate treatment, which can include creating music, singing, moving to music, or just listening to it (Achterberg et al., 1992).

The following procedures are used in music therapy:

- **Singing:** Helps individuals with speech impairments improve their articulation, rhythm, and breath control. For example, songs help elderly adults remember significant events in their lives.
- **Playing instruments:** Improves gross and fine motor coordination in individuals with motor impairments. For example, playing in an instrumental ensemble helps an individual with behavioral problems learn how to control disruptive impulses by working within a group structure.
- **Rhythmic movement:** Facilitates and improves an individual's range of motion, joint mobility, agility, strength, balance, coordination, gait consistency, respiration patterns, and muscular relaxation. For example, the rhythmic component of music helps to increase motivation, interest, and enjoyment, and it acts as a nonverbal persuasion to involve individuals socially.
- **Improvising:** Offers creative, nonverbal means of expressing feelings. For example, improvising offers an opportunity to make choices and deal with structure in a creative way.
- **Composing:** Develops cooperative learning and facilitates the sharing of feelings, ideas, and experiences. When used with hospitalized children, for example, writing songs provides an effective means of expressing and understanding fears.
- **Listening:** Used for many therapeutic applications, including the development of cognitive skills such as attention and memory. For example, actively listening to music in a relaxed and receptive state stimulates thoughts, images, and feelings, which can be further examined and discussed.

ART THERAPY

Art reflects the spiritual aspect of a person and brings harmony to the soul. As early as the 14th century, the Italians studied drawings made by individuals suffering from psychosis. The connection between art and mental health began to be recognized in the late 1800s with the advent of mental institutions (Achterberg et al., 1992; Tate & Longo, 2002).

Art is an expressive language that can enhance a relationship between client and provider by tapping into an individual's creativity and offering a nonthreatening form of communication over which the individual has control. The creative process of art can be a bridge to reconciling conflicts and increasing awareness. It can provide a permanent representation of an individual's internal states and can reflect changes seen in the therapeutic progression, provide graphic representation as opposed to verbalization, and increase expression and facilitate insight (Tate & Longo, 2002).

What Is Art Therapy?

Art therapy is a human service profession that utilizes art media, images, the creative art process, and client responses to create art productions as a reflection of the individual's development, abilities, personality, interests, concerns, and conflicts. The practice of art therapy is based on a knowledge of human developmental and psychological theories. Thoughts and feelings, metaphors, visualizations, and symbols can be expressed in more concrete and tangible ways through art therapy than through words alone (Perry, 2000; Tate & Longo, 2002).

Art therapy was formalized with the founding of the American Art Therapy Association in 1969. Today, art therapists must have a graduate degree and a strong foundation in the studio arts as well as in therapy techniques, and they must complete a supervised internship (Achterberg et al., 1992; Tate & Longo, 2002).

Art therapy differs from regular art classes such as painting, sculpting, and drawing because the therapist is trained in both diagnosis and in helping clients with specific health or spiritual problems. Art therapy stresses the process, not the product (Achterberg et al., 1992; Tate & Longo, 2002).

Therapeutic Effects and Benefits

Art therapy provides a way for clients to reconcile emotional conflicts, foster self-awareness, and express unspoken and frequently unconscious concerns about their disease. It is an effective treatment for the developmentally, medically, educationally, socially, or psychologically impaired. It is especially valuable with children, who often find it difficult to express their most painful concerns in more traditional therapeutic ways (Gabriel et al., 2001).

When used in psychosocial supportive interventions for cancer clients who were isolated for bone marrow transplantation, art therapy was shown to do the following (Gabriel et al., 2001):
- Strengthen their positive feelings
- Alleviate their distress
- Clarify their spiritual issues

The results of this study showed that art therapy may be especially beneficial for clients who need to deal with emotional conflicts and with feelings about life and death in a safe setting (Gabriel et al., 2001).

Art Therapy Interventions

Since they are trained in both art and therapy, art therapists are knowledgeable about human development, psychological theories, clinical practice, spirituality, multicultural and artistic traditions, and the healing potential of art.

Art is used by therapists in client treatment, assessment, and research, and when consulting with other allied health professionals. Working with people of all ages, races, and ethnic backgrounds, art therapists provide services, individually and as part of clinical teams, in a variety of settings, including the following (Gabriel et al., 2001; Perry, 2000; Rollins & Riccio, 2002):

- Psychiatric and medical hospitals and centers
- Drug and alcohol rehabilitation programs
- Medical and forensic institutions
- Correctional facilities
- Community outreach programs
- Wellness centers
- Schools
- Nursing homes and geriatric centers
- Senior centers
- Day-care treatment programs
- Corporate organizations
- Hospices
- Schools for the developmentally disabled
- Open studios
- Outpatient facilities
- Pain clinics
- Shelters
- Independent practices

Art Therapy Research

Research on art therapy has been conducted in clinical, educational, physiological, psychological, forensic, and sociological arenas. Studies on art therapy have been conducted in many clinical areas, including the following (Achterberg et al., 1992; Gabriel et al., 2001; Tate & Longo, 2002):

- Burn recovery in adolescent and young clients
- Eating disorders
- Emotional impairment in young children
- Reading performance
- Chemical addiction
- Cancer patients
- Mental illness
- As a prognostic aid in childhood cancer
- Bereavement
- Sexual abuse in adolescents
- Deafness, aphasia, autism, emotional disturbance, and brain injury in children

DANCE AND MOVEMENT THERAPY

Dance and movement are expressions of the mind, body, and spirit and are a powerful medium for therapy (Picard, 2000). A common thread in the vast array of theoretical orientations for dance and movement therapy is the focus on body movement as a manifestation of thoughts and feelings (Cohen & Walco, 1999). Dance is the essence of embodiment. An analysis of dance and movement provides an effective way of understanding the meaning of embodiment, which is defined as a way of being in a world of others (Block & Kissell, 2001).

Dance therapy began in the United States in 1942 through the pioneering efforts of Marian Chace. Psychiatrists found that their clients who attended her dance classes were receiving therapeutic benefits. As a result, Chace was asked to work with clients who had been considered too disturbed to participate in group activities (Achterberg et al., 1992).

In 1956, dance therapists founded the American Dance Therapy Association, which fosters research, monitors standards for professional practice, and develops guidelines for graduate education in dance therapy. Trained at the graduate level in dance and movement therapy, therapists take courses in psychopathology, psychotherapeutic theory, and human development and work with clients of all ages (Cotter, 1999).

Dance Therapy Goals and Interventions

Dance and movement therapists work with a variety of individuals in a variety of settings, and they address a diverse spectrum of disorders and disabilities. Dance and movement therapy incorporates an array of medical, psychological, social, and spiritual issues. Therapy goals and types of interventions vary according to the population served (Achterberg et al., 1992; Becker, 2002; Cohen & Walco, 1999; Peeke & Frishett, 2002; Picard, 2000; Rosler et al., 2002):

- For the emotionally disturbed, goals are to express feelings, gain insight, and develop attachments.
- For the physically disabled, goals are to increase movement and self-esteem, have fun, and heighten creativity.
- For the elderly, the goals are to maintain a healthy body, enhance vitality, develop relationships, enhance learning, develop some physical strength, and express fear and grief.
- For the mentally challenged, the goals are to motivate learning, increase body awareness, and develop social skills.

Dance therapy settings may include psychiatric centers, adult day-care facilities, community mental health centers, infant developmental centers, correctional facilities, schools, and rehabilitation facilities, as well as private practice outside an institution.

Benefits and Clinical Effectiveness of Dance Therapy

In many cultures of the world, dance plays an important role in healing and in health enhancement (Block & Kissell, 2001; Cotter, 1999). Dance and movement are used to prevent disease and to promote health for healthy people. They also reduce stress for caregivers and for patients with cancer, AIDS, and Alzheimer's disease (Achterberg et al., 1992; Cohen & Walco, 1999; Rosler et al., 2002).

The mind, body, and spirit are integrated in dance and movement therapy. As a result, it has been demonstrated to be clinically effective in achieving the following (Achterberg et al., 1992; Becker, 2002; Cohen & Walco, 1999; Picard, 2000):

- Developing an improved body image
- Improving self-concept
- Increasing self-esteem and self-awareness
- Facilitating attention
- Enhancing relationships with others, self, and spirit

- Ameliorating depression
- Decreasing fears and anxieties
- Expressing anger
- Decreasing feelings of isolation
- Improving communication skills
- Decreasing body tension
- Reducing chronic pain
- Enhancing circulatory and respiratory functions
- Promoting healing
- Increasing verbalization

Movement techniques such as yoga, Tai Chi, and Qi Gong may quiet the mind as well as aid in physical fitness and concentration. These techniques have meditative and spiritual qualities that provide the means to help a person experience the mind-body-spirit connection. In addition, the power of dance and movement can bring people together mentally, physically, and spiritually (Cohen & Walco, 1999; Picard, 2000).

HUMOR THERAPY

An Apache myth tells of how the creator endowed human beings,
the two-leggeds, with the ability to do everything—talk, run, see, and hear.
But he was not satisfied until the two-leggeds could do just one thing more—laugh. And
so men and women laughed and laughed and laughed!
Then the creator said, "Now you are fit to live."
—Larry Dossey (2001)

Humor is a universal and complex phenomenon. It is a holistic health practice that integrates physiologic, psychosocial, and spiritual well-being (Cohen, 1990). The culture, society, or ethnic group in which humor occurs influences its style and content as well as the situations in which it is used and is considered appropriate (Robinson, 1991; Ziv, 1988).

Studies have demonstrated that humor is a social relationship and occurs in a social environment. Humor promotes group cohesion, initiates relationships, relieves tension during social conflict, and can be a means of expressing approval or disapproval of social action (Wooten, 2000). Humor can stimulate the immune system, enhance perceptual flexibility, and renew spiritual energy (Wooten, 1996). In *Anatomy of an Illness*, Cousins (1979) describes how he used humor to help him recover from a debilitating disease. Many credit him as being the catalyst for a new specialty: humor therapy.

Humor and Laughter Defined

Before further discussion ensues, it is important to understand the definitions of humor and laughter. Wooten (2000) provides the following definitions:

- **Humor:** A quality of perception and attitude toward life that enables an individual to experience joy even when faced with adversity; a perception of the absurdity or incongruity of a situation.
- **Laughter:** A physical behavior that occurs in response to something perceived as humorous, amusing, or surprising. This behavior engages most of the mus-

cle groups and organ systems within the body. Laughter is often preceded by physical, emotional, or cognitive tension.

Humor is a complex concept, and three major theories of humor have arisen in an attempt to explain it (Dossey, 2001; Dossey et al., 2000; Robinson, 1991; Wooten, 2000):

1. The **incongruity theory** is considered a classic, traditional theory and considered by many to be a crucial component in the creation of humor. According to this theory, humor involves a sudden and surprising shift in an outcome one doesn't expect—where two concepts normally considered remote from each other are brought together to reveal their connection (e.g., the surprise ending of a joke).
2. The **release theory** describes the purpose or functions of humor. It claims that laughter occurs when the tension of anxiety or anger needs a release (e.g., nervous laughter).
3. The **superiority theory** is one of the oldest theories of humor. It is also a classic, traditional theory of humor that considers the element of assertion of one's superiority to be an ingredient in all humor. According to superiority theory, laughter comes from the enhanced feelings of self-esteem that occur in response to situations of others more unfortunate (e.g., seeing someone slip on ice).

Physiological Responses to Laughter

While humor is a perceptual process, laughter is a behavioral response. Laughter is a form of internal "jogging" that exercises the body and stimulates the release of beneficial brain neurotransmitters and hormones. Laughter is actually good for health, and it creates predictable, physiologic changes within the body. These occur within two stages of the body's response (Robinson, 1991; Wooten, 2000):

1. The **arousal stage**, in which physiologic parameters (i.e., heartbeat, pulse rate, blood pressure) increase.
2. The **resolution stage**, in which physiologic parameters return to resting values or lower.

Many muscle groups become active during laughter. These include the diaphragm; the abdominal, intercostal, respiratory accessory, and facial muscles; and sometimes muscles in the arms, legs, and back. During vigorous, sustained laughter, the heart rate is stimulated, normal respiratory patterns become chaotic, respiratory rate and depth are increased, and residual volume is decreased. Oxygen saturation of peripheral blood does not significantly change during the increased ventilation that occurs with laughter; therefore, conditions such as asthma or bronchitis may actually be aggravated by vigorous laughter.

Current research in the areas of psychology, physiology, and psychoneuroimmunology is defining the specific changes affected by the experience of mirthful laughter. Mirthful laughter has been shown to do the following (Berk, 1996; Wooten, 2000):

- Increase the number and activity of natural killer cells (which attack infected cells and some types of cancer cells).
- Increase the number of activated T cells (these cells are "turned on and ready to go" to fight infections).

- Increase the level of the antibody IgA (which fights upper respiratory tract infections).
- Increase the levels of gamma interferon (which activates many immune components).
- Increase levels of complement (which helps antibodies to pierce infected cells).

Laughter and Stress

The harmful effects of stress upon an individual's health are well known. Diseases such as hypertension, insomnia, ulcerative colitis, and coronary heart disease are, in part, the result of prolonged stress. Stress and negative emotions have been associated with immunosuppression and partially altered by increased epinephrine and cortisol blood levels.

The pleasant feelings associated with mirthful laughter may modify some of these neuroendocrine components of the stress response. In addition, there is a general decrease in stress hormones that constrict blood vessels and suppress immune activity after being exposed to humor (Berk, 1996).

Therapeutic Humor Interventions

Therapeutic humor has a beneficial effect on the mind, body, and spirit. There are three basic classifications of therapeutic humor: hoping humor, coping humor, and gallows humor (Dossey et al., 2000; Wooten, 2000).

- **Hoping humor:** Involves the ability to hope for something better that enables individuals to cope with difficult situations. Hoping humor accepts life with all its dichotomies, contradictions, and incongruities. It gives individuals the courage to withstand suffering.
- **Coping humor:** Involves laughing at hopeless situations. It provides a detachment from the problem and makes it possible to release tension, anxiety, and hostility.
- **Gallows humor:** Provides protection from the emotional impact of witnessing tragedy, disgusting or intolerable aspects of a situation, death, and disfigurement. Caregivers often use gallows humor as a means of maintaining some psychological distance from the suffering, thus protecting themselves from a sympathetic nervous system response to that suffering.

Health care and spiritual care providers can utilize therapeutic humor by incorporating humor and laughter into the clinical setting. Clients can be provided with many opportunities to laugh. Health care providers can offer humor in various formats (audio, video, reading, visual, and tactile) based on individual needs. These formats can involve any or all of the following (Cohen, 1990; Wooten, 2000):

- Discussing new research showing that humor and positive emotions facilitate recovery and enhance immune system function.
- Telling jokes (be sure the material is tasteful and appropriate for the client's age, gender, and culture; sexual, religious, or ethnic jokes should be avoided).
- Sharing cartoons and creating a scrapbook.
- Creating a bulletin board and posting cartoons, bumper stickers, and funny signs.

- Developing a file of funny jokes, stories, cards, bumper stickers, poems, and songs.
- Wearing a funny button, nose, or hat.
- Creating a humor journal or log to record funny encounters or humorous discoveries.
- Collecting funny books, videotapes, and audiotapes of comedy routines and creating a lending library.
- Forming an interdisciplinary humor committee of interested people who appreciate and use humor.
- Creating a "comedy cart" (a mobile unit with humor supplies), a humor room (a place where clients, families, and staff can gather to laugh, play, and relax together), or a humor basket (a small collection of comedy toys, gadgets, and props).

When therapeutic humor is used, it may reduce stress, boost immunity, relieve pain, decrease anxiety, stabilize mood, enhance communication, enhance self-esteem, and inspire creativity (Wooten, 2000). Cohen (1990) summarizes the therapeutic benefits of humor this way: "It is the overlapping nature of the physiological, psychological, social, and cognitive functions of humor that lead to healing and health, stress prevention and alleviation, pain management, higher self-esteem, improved relationships, and creative problem-solving" (p. 4).

ANIMAL-ASSISTED THERAPY

Throughout history, the bond between humans and animals has been clear. Both domesticated and wild animals have played a significant role in the lives of humans for thousands of years (Brodie & Biley, 1999). An example of this bond is animal-assisted therapy (AAT).

Over the past few decades, AAT has gained widespread support and application. It is defined as the utilization of animals as a therapeutic modality to facilitate healing and rehabilitation of clients with disabilities or acute or chronic ailments. While these programs have been called pet-assisted therapy, pet-facilitated therapy, pet therapy, animal-assisted activity, and animal visitation, animal-assisted therapy is the preferred term for a goal-directed intervention in which an animal that meets specific criteria is an integral part of the treatment process. Cognitive, physical, psychosocial, and spiritual benefits of AAT have been shown to include increased attention, orientation, and mobility (Cole & Gawlinski, 2000; Connor & Miller, 2000).

AAT is directed and/or delivered by health care professionals with specialized expertise and within the scope of practice of their profession into clients' treatment plans (Barker & Pandurangi, 2003). This differs from the main goal of a pet visitation program, which is primarily socialization (Connor & Miller, 2000). During AAT, the handler and the client's health care provider work together to develop specific clinical goals and interventions for the client and plans for how these goals will be accomplished. AAT is an interdisciplinary approach to care and an effective alternative therapeutic modality that can be used to promote quality of life and positive health benefits (Cole & Gawlinski, 2000; Khan & Farrag, 2000).

Theories on Animal-Assisted Therapy

Several theories attempt to explain the therapeutic effects of human interactions with therapy animals. The following summary provides an overview of three of these theories: social theory, therapeutic theory, and biophilic theory (Graham, 2000).

- **Social theory:** Advocates that human-animal interaction is influenced by differing cultures and should be viewed within a distinct social and environmental framework.
- **Therapeutic theory:** Argues that animals may be of therapeutic value in three general ways:
  1. As instruments helping individuals with special needs (i.e., guide dogs). Animals are an extension of the individual and provide an opportunity for control, increased coordination, mobility, and skill, resulting in improved confidence and self-esteem.
  2. Through passive involvement (e.g., gazing at fish in an aquarium or watching kittens at play). This method involves the individual being so absorbed in the animal's activity that relaxation results. The benefits are short-term and last as long as the animal is being observed.
  3. Through bonding and relationship. Anthropomorphic proponents suggest that the therapeutic effects of pet companions relate to the bonding potential between the animal and the owner and depend on the individual perceiving the animal as having human qualities. The animal's behavior is seen as expressing attachment, love, and devotion to the person and thus makes the person feel respected, loved, and needed by others. Animal therapy of this kind is most beneficial to individuals who feel unloved, socially alienated, friendless, or rejected.
- **Biophilic theory:** Proposes that animals offer a means for the estranged human to reconnect with the natural universe. Biophilia literally means "love of life." Biophilic theory proposes that a connection with nature is healthy and therapeutic on multiple levels. For example, it stimulates endorphins and boosts the immune system.

The Benefits of Animal-Assisted Therapy

The therapeutic effects of animals are diverse. Consider the following examples:

- Nutritional intake in individuals with Alzheimer's disease increases with the use of fish aquariums in the environment (Edwards & Beck, 2002).
- Stroking animals can relieve stress and depression (Brodie & Biley, 1999).
- Heart rate and blood pressure responses to acute stress were moderated by the mere presence of a pet in the room (Stanley-Hermanns & Miller, 2002).
- Clients with psychotic disorders and mood disorders had significant reductions in anxiety after AAT sessions (Stanley-Hermanns & Miller, 2002).
- The introduction of a friendly dog into a therapy session was associated with an increase in prosocial behavior and a decrease in autistic behavior in children (Martin & Farnum, 2002).
- Pets supply ongoing comfort and reduce feelings of loneliness during life crises or stressful transitions such as divorce or bereavement (Brodie & Biley, 1999).

- Pet owners experience significantly reduced cholesterol and blood fat levels and dramatically improved postmyocardial infarction survival rates compared to nonpet owners (Brodie & Biley, 1999).
- Interacting with and caring for pets improves a client's strength, endurance, range of motion, balance, mobility, and sensation (Duncan, 2000).

In addition, AAT offers several other therapeutic benefits, including the following.

Animals and Communication

Therapy animals are nonjudgmental, offer unconditional love, and make it easier for individuals (such as residents in long-term care and hospice facilities) to talk with each other by providing a point of common interest on which to focus a conversation. Animals can also help build rapport between the client and the health care provider (Connor & Miller, 2000).

Many individuals in hospitals or group homes had pets in the past and miss the companionship a pet provides. A visit with a therapy animal can evoke pleasant memories, reduce loneliness, and provide the opportunity for unconditional acceptance. These benefits last long after the therapy animal has gone home (Banks & Banks, 2002).

Animals and Social Support

Social support has an important influence on an individual's health, and pets may act as providers of social support (Brodie & Biley, 1999). Graham (2000) defines social support as "social, emotional, and instrumental exchanges with which the individual is involved, having the . . . consequence that an individual sees him or herself as an object of continuing value in the eyes of significant others" (p. 53).

Social support is important in the recovery of a wide range of medical conditions and stressful life events. According to Graham (2000, pp. 54-55), pets may provide social support in three ways:

1. Pets are perceived as always available, predictable in their responses, and non-judgmental.
2. No social skills are required to obtain their approval, thus removing the potential problem of how to ask for or elicit support.
3. Pets may provide a refuge from the strains of human interactions, provide breathing space, and provide an opportunity for naturalness that is particularly relaxing.

Animals and Individuals With Disabilities

Individuals with a traumatic brain injury, those who have suffered strokes, or those with a severe physical impairment may suffer dramatic changes to their personal appearance, independence, mobility, and cognitive functioning.

Therapy animals can play a critical role in helping these individuals improve their self-esteem and well-being. For example, spinal cord injury patients experienced reduced stress, increased self-esteem, improved communication, and increased sensory stimulation during animal therapy sessions (Counsell, Abram, & Gilbert, 1997).

Events that might be considered stressful or insurmountable to these individuals often become much more manageable after AAT sessions. Pets in the home and therapy animals often make it possible for these individuals to enter college, become employed, make friends, use fewer health care services, and become more independent.

Types of Therapy Animals

Therapy animals fall into four major classifications: service, therapy, social, and companion animals (Cole & Gawlinski, 2000; Connor & Miller, 2000; Duncan, 2000; Huebscher, 2000; Jorgenson, 1997; Laun, 2003).

Service Animals

A service animal is defined as any animal individually trained to do work or perform tasks for the benefit of a person with a disability. Dogs are the animals most commonly used for these tasks, which can include the following:

- Guiding a person who is sight impaired
- Pulling a wheelchair
- Assisting a person with impaired hearing
- Retrieving items

Service animals are not considered pets because they are trained to meet the specific disability-related needs of their owners. Federal laws protect the rights of individuals to have their service animals accompany them in public places if they meet the definition of having a disability.

According to the Americans with Disabilities Act, an individual is considered to be disabled if he or she meets at least one of the following tests:

- Having a physical or mental impairment that substantially limits one or more major life activities
- Having a record of such an impairment
- Being regarded as having such an impairment

Therapy Animals

Federal law does not define therapy animals, although some state laws define them. Therapy animals are usually the personal pets of their handlers, are used to provide opportunities for people to be in contact with animals, and may be used to work with individuals with disabilities. Federal laws do not protect people accompanied by their therapy animals in public places with a "no pets" policy. Therapy animals are not service animals.

The use of pets as therapy animals is a centuries-old treatment program dating back to the 9th century AD in Belgium, when animals were used in caring for individuals with disabilities. Pet therapy (the use of pets as therapy animals) is now being validated via scientific and anecdotal data to confirm its effectiveness. Medical and mental health programs around the world are using animals in treatment programs (Laun, 2003).

Social Animals

Social animals are those animals that did not complete a service animal training program due to temperament, health, training, or other problems, but they are made available as pets to individuals with disabilities.

Companion Animals

Companion animal is another term for "pet." There are no legal definitions for these animals at this time. Companion animals can include an individual's personal pet, pets used in AAT, and pets that actually "live" in a medical setting (Donowitz, 2002).

Animals That Heal

While many types of pets, including rabbits, birds, and horses, are suitable for AAT, dogs and cats are the most commonly used, perhaps due to the special relationship humans have developed with them through centuries of domestication. Whichever type of animal is chosen, AAT can act as a catalyst to make other traditional therapies (such as physical therapy, psychotherapy, or occupational therapy) more effective.

Therapy With Dogs

Dogs are by far the most commonly used animals in AAT. They guide people who are visually impaired, hear for those who are hearing impaired, predict seizures in epileptic patients, and perform a myriad of duties for those who are disabled. Dogs are a natural choice for AAT programs because humans have had a deep and intimate relationship with dogs for centuries; because of their calm, nonjudgmental nature; and because of their ability to provide unconditional support and acceptance.

When people learned that more than 7,000 British, American, and German dogs were killed in action during World War I, they quickly realized the vital service these animals could provide. The use of service dogs in a variety of ways soon followed (Graham, 2000):

- The Germans, during the 1920s, were the first to train dogs to lead blind people.
- Hearing Dogs for Deaf People was established in 1982.
- Pets as Therapy Dogs started in 1983 in recognition of the numbers of people who lacked contact with animals.
- Dogs for the Disabled was established in 1986.
- Support Dogs was set up in 1992 to assist owners with specific disabilities (such as seizures).
- Canine Partners for Independence (CPI) trains dogs to respond to over 90 verbal commands (such as opening and shutting doors, fetching items, picking up dropped items, drawing the curtains, and taking laundry out of a washing machine).

Today, the use of dogs in AAT is global, and dog therapy programs continue to be some of the most effective forms of AAT.

Therapy With Cats

Due to their independent nature, cats are used less frequently than dogs as therapy animals. Visiting cat programs currently appear to be rather rare, but the number of cats kept as pets is steadily increasing (Graham, 2000). Cats are quickly becoming the companion animals of choice for those individuals who are not at home during the day.

Cat owners have significantly better general psychological health than nonpet owning individuals, but it is rare for cats to offer the practical support and assistance that dogs can (Graham, 2000). However, caressing and stroking cats provides an opportunity for touching and physical contact that can be extremely important to an individual's sense of well-being.

Therapy With Horses

Because horses are highly sensitive and responsive, they make excellent therapy animals. The social support obtained from a horse is unlike that of most other animals. Horses are unable to share a human living environment, but they provide comfort, solace, and nonjudgmental encounters. Because of a horse's sheer size and power, clients who are involved in therapy programs with them experience feelings of tremendous achievement, self-worth, and self-esteem.

Hippotherapy is one particular type of therapy program involving horses. This type of AAT literally means treatment with the help of a horse and refers to the spiritual, physical, and psychological benefits derived from riding a horse (Vidrine, Owen-Smith, & Faulkner, 2002). Hippotherapy is an integrated therapy program involving the development of long- and short-term goals for the client (Jorgenson, 1997).

Classic hippotherapy has been widely practiced in Europe since the 1960s. It usually involves a specially trained physical therapist, occupational therapist, or speech language pathologist who focuses the training on the rider's posture and movement responses as well as on other psychological, cognitive, social, spiritual, behavioral, and communicative goals.

Therapeutic riding influences the whole person, and the effect on many of the body systems can be profound. Any riding program using horse-related activities for clients with physical, spiritual, mental, cognitive, social, or behavioral problems is a therapeutic riding program.

Animal-Assisted Therapy Settings

AAT is effective in many environments. Trained volunteers and staff with two- and four-legged therapists visit individuals in all sorts of places, including the following (Connor & Miller, 2000):

- Nursing homes
- Mental health care units
- Residential treatment centers
- Senior day-care centers
- Long-term care facilities
- Schools for the disabled
- Hospice care centers
- Correctional facilities
- Acute care and intensive care units
- Oncology units
- Clients' homes
- Psychiatric facilities
- Speech and occupational units

SUMMARY

The mind-body-spirit therapeutic interventions of music, art, dance, humor, and AAT can be integrated into mainstream medicine and should be considered as complements to mainstream medical treatments, not as a replacement for them. The National Center for Complementary and Alternative Medicine (NCCAM) is evaluating these therapies, and research is demonstrating that these therapeutic interventions are not only safe but effective as well.

KEY CONCEPTS

1. Music therapy as a spiritual dimension is a powerful holistic method of healing used successfully with people of all ages and disabilities.
2. Art therapy is effective in strengthening positive feelings, alleviating distress, and clarifying spiritual issues.
3. Dance therapy is an expression of the mind-body-spirit and incorporates an array of medical, psychological, social, and spiritual issues.
4. Humor therapy is a holistic health practice that integrates physiologic, psychosocial, and spiritual well-being.
5. AAT is an interdisciplinary approach to care that utilizes animals as a therapeutic modality to facilitate healing and rehabilitation of clients with disabilities or acute or chronic ailments.

QUESTIONS FOR REFLECTION

1. What are some of the ways you use therapeutic interventions to enhance your own spirituality? For example, do you play music to elevate your mood or relax after a rough day? Do you send and receive jokes and funny stories over the Internet?
2. If you don't have access to some of the formalized therapeutic interventions listed here, what are some ways you could introduce these methods to your patients or clients?

REFERENCES

Achterberg, J., Dossey, B., & Kolkmeir, L. (1994). *Rituals of healing: Using imagery for health and wellness.* New York: Bantam Books.

Achterberg, J., Dossey, L., Gordon, J. S., Hegedus, C., Herrmann, M. W., & Nelson, R. (1992). *Mind-body interventions.* In BM Berman & DB Larson (Eds.), *Alternative medicine: Expanding medical horizons. (A report to the National Institutes of Health on alternative medical systems and practices in the United States).* Chantilly, VA: U.S. Government Printing Office.

Banks, M. R., & Banks, W. A. (2002). The effects of animal-assisted therapy on loneliness in an elderly population in long-term care facilities. *Journal of Gerontology, Series A: Biological Sciences and Medical Sciences, 57*(7), 428-432.

Barker, S. B., & Pandurangi, A. K. (2003). Effects of animal-assisted therapy on patients' anxiety, fear, and depression before ECT. *Journal of ECT, 19*(1), 38-44.

Becker, B. (2002). Stage presence—body presence: Movement and body experience with the elderly. *Case Management Journals, 3*(2), 99-106.

Berk, L. (1996). The laughter-immune connection: New discoveries. *Humor and Health Journal, 5*(5), 1-7.

Block, B., & Kissell, J. L. (2001). The dance: Essence of embodiment. *Theoretical Medicine and Bioethics, 22*(1), 5-15.

Brodie, S. J., & Biley, F. C. (1999). An exploration of the potential benefits of pet-facilitated therapy. *Journal of Clinical Nursing, 8*(4), 329-337.

Cabrera, I. N., & Lee, M. H. (2000). Reducing noise pollution in the hospital setting by establishing a department of sound: A survey of recent research on the effects of noise and music in health care. *Preventive Medicine, 30,* 339-349.

Campbell, D. (2001). *The Mozart effect.* New York: HarperCollins.

Cohen, M. (1990). Caring for ourselves can be funny business. *Holistic Nursing Practice, 4*(4), 1-11.

Cohen, S. O., & Walco, G. A. (1999). Dance/movement therapy for children and adolescents with cancer. *Cancer Practice, 7*(1), 34-42.

Cole, K. M., & Gawlinski, A. (2000). Animal-assisted therapy: The human-animal bond. *AACN Clinical Issues, 11*(1), 139-149.

Connor, K., & Miller, J. (2000). Animal-assisted therapy: An in-depth look. *Dimensions of Critical Care, 19*(3), 20-26.

Cotter, A. C. (1999). Western movement therapies. *Physical Medicine and Rehabilitation Clinics of North America, 10*(3), 603-615.

Counsell, C. M., Abram, J., & Gilbert, M. (1997). Animal-assisted therapy and the individual with spinal cord injury. *SCI Nurse, 4*(2), 52-55.

Cousins, N. (1979). *Anatomy of an illness.* New York: W. W. Norton.

Donowitz, L. G. (2002). Pet therapy. *Pediatric Infectious Disease Journal, 21*(1), 64-66.

Dossey, L. (2001). *Healing beyond the body: Medicine and the infinite reach of the mind.* Boston: Shambhala.

Dossey, B. M., Keegan, L., & Guzzetta, C. E. (2000). *Holistic nursing: A handbook for practice* (3rd ed.). Gaithersburg, MD: Aspen.

Duncan, S. L. (2000). APIC state-of-the art report: The implications of service animals in health care settings. *American Journal of Infection Control, 28*(2), 170-180.

Edwards, N. E., & Beck, A. M. (2002). Animal-assisted therapy and nutrition in Alzheimer's disease. *Western Journal of Nursing Research, 24*(6), 697-712.

Gabriel, B., Bromberg, E., Vandenbovenkamp, J., Walka, P., Kornblith, A. B., & Luzzatto, P. (2001). Art therapy with adult bone marrow transplant patients in isolation: A pilot study. *Psychooncology, 10*(2), 114-123.

Graham, B. (2000). *Creature comfort: Animals that heal.* New York: Prometheus Books.

Huebscher, R. (2000). Pets and animal-assisted therapy. *Nurse Practitioner Forum, 11*(1), 1-4.

Jorgenson, J. (1997). Therapeutic use of companion animals in health care. *Image: Journal of Nursing Scholarship, 29*(3), 249-254.

Khan, M. A., & Farrag, N. (2000). Animal-assisted activity and infection control implications in a health care setting. *Journal of Hospital Infection, 46*(1), 4-11.

Laun, L. (2003). Benefits of pet therapy in dementia. *Home Healthcare Nurse, 21*(1), 49-52.

Martin, F., & Farnum, J. (2002). Animal-assisted therapy for children with pervasive developmental disorders. *Western Journal of Nursing Research, 24*(6), 657-670.

Matthews, D. A., & Clark, C. (1998). *The faith factor: Proof of the healing power of prayer.* New York: Penguin Books.

Peeke, P. M., & Frishett, S. (2002). The role of complementary and alternative therapies in women's mental health. *Primary Care: Clinics in Office Practice, 29*(1), 1-14.

Perry, R. C. (2000). Drawing from within: Art therapy can speak for—and heal—your residents. *Contemporary Long Term Care, 23*(11), 22-25.

Picard, C. (2000). Pattern of expanding consciousness in midlife women: Creative movement and the narrative as modes of expression. *Nursing Science Quarterly, 13*(2), 150-157.

Robinson, V. M. (1991). *Humor and the health professions: The therapeutic use of humor in health care.* Thorofare, NJ: SLACK Incorporated.

Rollins, J. A., & Riccio, L. L. (2002). ART is the heART: A palette of possibilities for hospice care. *Pediatric Nursing, 28*(4), 355-362.

Rosler, A., Seifritz, E., Krauchi, K., Spoerl, D., Brokkuslaus, I., Proserpi, S. M., et al. (2002). Skill learning in patients with moderate Alzheimer's disease: A prospective pilot study. *International Journal of Geriatric Psychiatry, 17*(12), 1155-1156.

Schroeder-Sheker, T. (1994). Music for the dying: A personal account of the new field of music-thanatology—history, theories, and clinical narratives. *Journal of Holistic Nursing, 12*(1), 83-99.

Stanley-Hermanns, M., & Miller, J. (2002). Animal-assisted therapy. *American Journal of Nursing, 102*(10), 69-76.

Tate, F. B., & Longo, D. A. (2002). Art therapy: Enhancing psychosocial nursing. *Journal of Psychosocial Nursing, 40*(3), 40-47.

Taylor, E. J. (2002). *Spiritual care.* Upper Saddle River, NJ: Prentice Hall.

Updike, P. A. (1998). Opening to the sacred: Intentional use of music to engage the spiritual dimension. *Advanced Practice Nursing, 4*(1), 64-69.

Vidrine, M., Owen-Smith, P., & Faulkner, P. (2002). Equine-facilitated group psychotherapy: Applications for therapeutic vaulting. *Issues in Mental Health Nursing, 23*(6), 587-603.

Wooten, P. (1996). Humor: An antidote for stress. *Holistic Nursing Practice, 10*(2), 49-56.

Wooten, P. (2000). Humor, laughter, and play: Maintaining balance in a serious world. In B. M. Dossey, L. Keegan, & C. E. Guzzetta (Eds.), *Holistic nursing: A handbook for practice* (3rd ed., pp. 471-493). Gaithersburg, MD: Aspen.

Ziv, A. (1988). *National styles of humor.* Westport, CT: Greenwood.

8

SPIRITUALLY HEALING ENVIRONMENTS

*"We need the tonic of the wilderness...
we can never have enough of nature."*
—Henry David Thoreau

LEARNING OBJECTIVES

Upon completing this course, you will be able to do the following:
1. Define *healing environment*.
2. Identify outcomes of healing environments.
3. Describe the roles of color, nature, and lighting in creating a spiritually healing environment.
4. Describe the roles of air quality, temperature, and smells in a spiritually healing environment.
5. Describe the roles of music, noise, and furnishings in a spiritually healing environment.
6. Define *wayfinding* and describe its importance in a healthy environment.
7. Explain the role of the health care provider in creating a spiritually healing environment.

INTRODUCTION

Florence Nightingale, the founder of modern nursing, was one of the first individuals to realize the impact of lighting, noise, and sensory stimulation on healing. She strongly believed that nature alone cures and the role of nursing is to put the patient in the best possible situation for nature to act (Fontaine, Briggs, & Pope-

Smith, 2001; Stichler, 2001). During her care of the patients in British hospitals after the Crimean War, she fought for calm, airy, nature-oriented rooms filled with colorful art (Weber, 1996). Ms. Nightingale was one of the first health care professionals to realize the impact of the environment on the patient's ability to heal. She was also one of the first individuals to explore, and document, the health care professional's role in incorporating nature and the environment in such a way that patients could begin their healing journey.

Health care providers have the power to create a spiritually healing environment that allows clients to access their "inner healer"—that phenomenon of healing that transcends social, cultural, economic, time, and space barriers and promotes healing. Healthy environments and sacred spaces are powerful ways to support the inner healer and utilize the environment to maximize its healing effects. When a building is well designed, it brings a natural and organic energy as well as a spirituality to the environment (Long, 2001; Stichler, 2001; Wright & Sayre-Adams, 2000). However, though good facility design is important, health care organizations do not have to remodel to create a specific environment. How clients are treated and how staff treat one another is perhaps the most important component of a healing environment ("Healing Environments," 2002).

WHAT IS A SPIRITUALLY HEALING ENVIRONMENT?

In its broadest sense, the term *environment* can mean everything within as well as external to an individual. Environments and spaces are much more than locations. They contain memories, experiences, energy, and meaning (Hasselkus, 2002). A *spiritually healing environment* is one in which individuals are supported and nurtured, in which they feel spiritually calm, and in which health and well-being are promoted. Healing environments play a vital role in maintaining a healthy lifestyle and are just as important as eating properly, exercising regularly, practicing proper health care, and having meaningful relationships and support systems. Spiritually healing environments promote a sense of relaxation and peace, and they help to vitalize senses that may have been dulled (Spalding, 2001).

Spiritually healing environments are quality spaces with adequate room, proper plumbing, clean indoor water sources, low levels of ambient noise, and safe surroundings (Evans & Kantrowitz, 2002). According to Neumann and Mensik (1993), "Healing institutions integrate sensitive and compassionate care, a nurturing environment, and healing modalities as well as curing into their patients' overall experience" (p. 2).

Many people may not even notice the effects the environment may have on them. They are so familiar with working in conditions that are cold, lacking in natural light, and filled with artificial energies that they become accustomed to them. Individuals living in Western society often live a "disconnected" existence. For example, many work environments do not allow for windows to be open to fresh air, and houses are built on tiny lots with no open space or room for local wildlife. Health care environments are often painted in cold tones and filled with unfamiliar, stressful noises and smells. This disconnection from the natural world can leave people feeling estranged and unfulfilled. They may feel stressed and seek artificial substitutes for natural experiences.

Human beings are intimately connected to planet Earth. They share the planet with every other living organism and they are just one strand in the complex web of life. When they live a disconnected existence, they become unhealthy, unbalanced, and unhappy. Yet, when they are in a healing environment, they know it. They feel welcome, balanced, relaxed, reassured, and stimulated (Stichler, 2001).

Spiritually healing environments are healthy environments. They connect people with nature and natural elements that contribute to their health and well-being. They are filled with individuals who care for themselves and for each other in a compassionate way. These environments allow a greater sense of control. They provide privacy; enhance a connection with nature, culture, and people; provide vital social support; provide appropriate activities and distractions; and provide people with the ability to cope more effectively with stress. Healing spaces are spiritual places with "heightened meaning and keen personal significance" (Hasselkus, 2002, p. 33). They are a crucial element of healing.

A Shift in Focus

The relationship between the mind, body, spirit, nature, and healing has been demonstrated for many centuries by many cultures. Neumann and Mensik (1993) provide several examples:

- **The ancient Greeks** worshipped the god of healing by building healing temples among cypress groves near the ocean. They faced the ocean and took advantage of the sea breezes and the sun. Patients at the temples used libraries, gardens, baths, theaters, gymnasiums, and special sleep rooms to heal. They took part in activities specially designed to restore their natural body rhythms, thus achieving harmony between their body and their mind.
- **The ancient Egyptians** decorated their healing places with murals because they believed the murals helped patients maintain their interest in life.
- **Early Christians** designed their hospitals after cathedrals so patients would feel confident, spiritual, serene, and strong.
- **Various European and Asian groups** have embraced holistic healing through the use of light therapy, music, nutrition, and herbs.
- **Native Americans** believe in the sacredness of special places. They believe that a state of good health results from harmony and balance with the physical, social, and spiritual aspects of life (Rose, 1993).

Yet, for much of the 19th and 20th centuries in the United States, no clear attention was paid to this relationship except by a very few individuals. Instead, Americans focused on specific environmental concerns.

Hospital design began to undergo a complete evolution in the 1970s when consumers started to consider aesthetic appeal as a major determinant in choosing a hospital for care. Maternity wards were the first to be renovated, since hospital executives realized that women had the time and the power to make a choice about where to deliver their babies. The results were so dramatic that other units began to renovate their environments to better appeal to the patients who would be healing there (Stichler, 2001).

Today, health care organizations and health care professionals are committed to providing healthy, healing environments for their clients. In 1984, Roger Ulrich discovered that postsurgical patients recovered more quickly when their hospital rooms offered a view of the outside world. He helped pioneer a new area of science that studies the interaction between the environment and healing. This area of study has been called supportive, evidence-informed, or research-based design (Bilchik, 2002). An additional concept that is still being studied is that of biophilia, which proposes that human beings are evolutionarily "hardwired" to respond in a visceral manner to their surroundings and that this trait has contributed to our survival as a species. Infants, for example, still respond with a startle reflex when they hear a loud noise in their environment (Bilchik, 2002).

By increasing their awareness of environmental issues and holistic health care practices, health care professionals contribute to the movement toward healthy healing environments. Many organizations have shifted their philosophy to reflect the concept that technology mends while compassion heals, so that world-class health care can be delivered in environments that are comfortable, healing, and humane (Martineck, 2001). Research has contributed to this effort by demonstrating the impact of health care environments and processes on a variety of factors, from nosocomial infections to stress and staff turnover (Bilchik, 2002). For example, in 1999, JCAHO published major revisions in its hospital accreditation manual that rates health care organizations on their ability to provide a healing environment for their staff and clients. These new JCAHO guidelines do not outline what changes need to be made; instead, they allow organizations to identify their own areas for improvement (Garber, 1999).

Increasingly, sicker clients challenge health care organizations to provide a higher level of care and to be more outcome oriented and more cost conscious in their delivery of care. At the same time, a paradigm shift in health care delivery is also taking place. The traditional medical model of trying to cure diseases is being replaced by a more holistic approach that involves healing the whole client. The creation of healing environments is a natural outgrowth of the centuries-old concept of mind-body healing, the environmental movement in the United States, recent studies in environmental psychology, and holistic practices (Neumann & Mensik, 1993).

Increasing data indicate that clients experience a positive outcome in an environment that incorporates natural light, natural elements, soothing colors, meaningful and varying stimuli, less noise, natural views, and a sense of beauty (Stichler, 2001). Yet, with the pressure that managed care has exerted on the budgets of most health care facilities, many are spending much less on infrastructure, resulting in newer buildings that are often lower in quality than the older buildings were (Weber, 1996).

THE POWER OF DESIGN

> U.S. health care institutions are... staff intensive. Patient outcomes are suffering... Managed care needs... health-care models that improve patent outcomes, lower liability, and reduce costs... [E]mpowering design details can reduce costs as patients take responsibilities for their health care and decrease their reliance on staff. (Leibrock, 2000, pp. xv-xvi)

According to Leibrock (2000), "without these details, health care facilities are places where patients are overexposed to strangers and separated from family, where independence is lost to providers or to disabling design" (p. xvi).

Good design is cost effective and improves staff retention (Domrose, 2002; Ulrich, 2002; Voelker, 2001). Effectively designed health care settings can nurture, comfort, relax, strengthen, and add to a sense of well-being. As hospitals and health care facilities transform their high-tech environments into comfortable, more user-friendly spaces, clients and their families will be supported and empowered in their healing journey (Neumann & Mensik, 1993).

CREATING A SPIRITUALLY HEALING ENVIRONMENT

A spiritually healing environment can be created in an institutional or personal setting. The creation of a healing environment involves attention to specific design elements as well as cultural- and age-specific details. Spiritually healing environments engage all five senses. They maximize choice and independence and include attention to specific design details such as color, nature, lighting, air quality and temperature, smells, noise, music, furnishings, and wayfinding (Weber, 1996).

Color

Color has been an important part of spirituality and the healing process for thousands of years. The ancient Egyptians ascribed healing powers to various colors. The Indian culture assigns colors and specific meanings to the 12 chakras, or energy centers of the body. Archeologists have found that ancient temples were oriented in such a way that light shining through various openings created prisms of light that shone in special chambers used for healing the sick. Florence Nightingale used color as a healing therapy, primarily through the use of fresh flowers for her patients.

The effects of color on human behavior and the physiological systems of the body are well documented. Color has been shown to affect heart rates, brainwave activity, respirations, and muscular tension. Color has meaning to most individuals, and lack of color can be a source of stress. Color can make a space feel restful, cheerful, stimulating, or irritating. There are several guidelines about the use of color in health care environments. However, the needs of specific populations must be taken into consideration when using color to create healing spaces (Fontaine et al., 2001; Leibrock, 2000; Long, 2001; Neumann & Mensik, 1993).

Chromotherapy

A specific discipline called chromotherapy uses colors to treat individuals suffering from certain disorders (Fontaine et al., 2001).

- Warmer colors (such as peach, soft yellows, or coral) can stimulate the appetite and encourage alertness, creativity, and socialization; these colors are useful in such areas as dining rooms or meeting spaces.
- Blues, greens, violets, and other cool colors are useful in areas designed to be restful, spiritual, contemplative, and quiet (such as waiting rooms or meditation areas).
- Primary colors (red, yellow, and blue) and strong patterns are pleasing at first but can be overstimulating and may contribute to fatigue.
- Green symbolizes growth, healing, spirituality, and peace, and has been used to reduce tension and nervousness.
- The brain requires constant stimulation. Monotonous color schemes contribute to sensory deprivation, disorganization of brain function, deterioration of intelligence, and an inability to concentrate. They slow the healing process and are perceived as "institutional."
- Color affects an individual's perception of time, size, weight, and volume. For example, warm color schemes are better in rooms where pleasant activities (such as dining or recreation) take place, since the activity seems to last longer. In rooms where monotonous tasks are performed, a cool color scheme can make time pass more quickly.

Nature

All living creatures are influenced by the rhythms of seasonal change and by their own intrinsic rhythms. Much of how humans perceive this change is based on daily light cycles, the rising and setting of the sun, the yearly changes in length of day, and even the rhythms of the tides. Chronobiology, the cyclical view of time and rhythms and their effect on the body, is important in the design of patient rooms. (Neumann & Mensik, 1993, p. 4)

Natural elements, time spent in connection with nature, views of nature, and natural lighting can have a powerful effect on the healing process. For example, patients in rooms with views of nature heal faster and leave the hospital earlier than those patients whose rooms have no view or a poor view. Those who are exposed to a nature scene require less pain medication and sedation and have lower blood pressure (Bilchik, 2002; Fontaine et al., 2001; Neumann & Mensik, 1993). In one study, patients who saw a nature scene (either real or in a photograph or painting) and who listened to nature sounds were much less anxious and had improved cardiac oxygenation (Ulrich, 2002). Cancer patients respond positively to living, growing things in the environment, since they contain strong metaphors for life (Leibrock, 2000). Patients whose rooms overlooked vegetation recovered faster after gallbladder surgery and required less pain medication than those without a view of nature (Gilhooley & Rice, 2002).

"Nature fascination," "sensory joy," peacefulness, and tranquility are all feelings reported by those individuals who participate in gardening activities. Yet, few health care facilities today utilize gardens (Marcus & Barnes, 1995).

According to Marcus & Barnes (1995), the first restorative gardens in Europe occurred in the Middle Ages when hospitals and monasteries were used to care for the sick, the insane, and the infirm. These places often incorporated a courtyard that provided the residents with shelter, sunlight, or shade as well as sensory stimulation. This trend declined during the 14th and 15th centuries. By the 19th century, gardening and farming were used as therapeutic regimens in the treatment of the mentally ill. Finally, during the 20th century, the trend declined again with the development of high-rise construction and rapid advances in medical science. Air-conditioned offices and a "health care industry" stimulated competition for patients so that hospitals began to look like hotel lobbies or resorts. However, as complementary and alternative medicine is beginning to demonstrate the intimate relationship between the mind and the body, design professionals are beginning to rediscover the therapeutic possibilities of a well-planned garden and landscape.

Research shows that plants (and even a view of plants) lower people's stress levels, lower blood pressure, reduce muscle tension, and contribute significantly to healing (Gilhooley & Rice, 2002). This can contribute to a health care organization's bottom line. For example, plants enhance people's perception of a building and make them feel more welcome and relaxed—two important conditions for patients and families. This may, in turn, attract more patients, contribute to employee retention, and lift the spirits of everyone in the environment (Gilhooley & Rice, 2002).

Lighting

Light is "a form of electromagnetic energy that can have both positive and negative effects on living organisms" (Fontaine et al., 2001, p. 24). It can affect human beings in a variety of ways (Fontaine et al., 2001; Higgins, 2002; McColl & Veitch, 2001; Wallace-Guy et al., 2002):

- Light absorption through the skin stimulates chemical reactions in the blood and tissues, such as that seen with vitamin D synthesis (important in decreasing osteoporosis and bone fractures).
- Light absorption by the skin produces both protective and pathological responses.
- Light exposure can be used to treat hyperbilirubinemia in neonates.
- Ultraviolet radiation can positively and negatively affect the immune system functioning in animals and humans.
- Full-spectrum fluorescent lamps (FSFL) may affect hormone secretion, physical activity levels, and performance; cause fewer headaches; and result in less stress.
- Light therapy is effective in reducing depressive mood disorders, eating disorders that are affected by the seasons, jet lag, shift work disorders, and premenstrual dysphoria.
- Light can affect sleep and modulate the body's corticosteroid and thyroid hormone levels.

The Benefits of Ultraviolet Light

Ultraviolet light is part of the electromagnetic spectrum and is a form of short-wave radiation invisible to the human eye. The earth's atmosphere effectively blocks the transmission of most ultraviolet light. According to Stichler (2001), ultraviolet light can do the following:
- Increase protein metabolism
- Lessen fatigue
- Stimulate white blood cell production
- Increase the release of endorphins
- Lower blood pressure
- Elevate mood
- Promote emotional well-being

As individuals age, their experience of the light around them changes. Their eyes may adjust to light more slowly or they may be unable to distinguish changes in light levels. Sensitivity to glare increases, and lenses may undergo a yellow tinting that affects the way color is perceived. Depth perception may be altered and peripheral vision may decrease (Leibrock, 2000). Individuals who are ill or stressed often experience disorientation, which can be decreased by effective lighting.

In addition, exposure to artificial light has been implicated in breast cancer (Hansen, 2001; Schernhammer et al., 2001). Artificial light is believed to suppress the normal nocturnal production of melatonin by the pineal gland. Melatonin is a hormone that helps regulate the body's circadian rhythms and sleep. In several studies, low melatonin levels have been linked to cancer growth. While this area of research needs to be studied further before any final conclusions can be drawn, these initial results are alarming. According to Hansen (2001), "No occupational exposures with known or potential carcinogenicity are as common as work at night" (p. 1513). Since society has increased the diversity of work hours, including working at night and shift work, the effect of light on health must be explored.

Taking these and other concerns into consideration, lighting is an important design feature for health and safety. Fluorescent lighting, and its possible effects on health, mood, and behavior, is of particular concern in the design of healing environments. While natural daylight is believed to be best for health, many individuals live and work in environments lit by fluorescent lighting. FSFL have been designed as an alternative to traditional fluorescent lighting. They mimic the spectral qualities of daylight and provide similar health-promoting effects to those of natural light. The principle behind the development of FSFL is that since life evolved around daylight, optimal physiological functioning will continue under this type of light and any deviation from it might lead to less-than-optimal functioning. However, while much of the public accepts these alleged health benefits, they remain controversial (McColl & Veitch, 2001).

Guidelines for incorporating healthy lighting features into a healing environment include the following (Fontaine et al., 2001; Leibrock, 2000; Long, 2001):
- Keep lighting levels consistent and adjustable from space to space.
- Utilize windows for the natural light and views they provide. Vertical blinds and other window treatments allow light intensity to be adjusted as needed.

- Use night lights in bedrooms and corridors. Install lights near bed perimeters or on nightstands for easy access.
- Since many accidents occur in the bathroom, lighting must be appropriate (without glare) and sufficient. Steam-filled showers, for example, may decrease visibility. Vapor-proof light fixtures in the ceiling of shower stalls and exhaust fans are important features that reduce steam and improve visibility.
- Prevent contrast glare by using shields or frosted globes on lights. Matte finishes for furniture, fixtures, and equipment also help to reduce glare.
- Sufficient lighting should be provided in areas requiring concentration, decision making, or areas of potential danger.
- Install dimmers on light switches to reduce glare.
- Eliminate glare on computer screens by using a nonglare fixture.
- Use lighting with spectrums as close to daylight as possible. This can reduce depression, fatigue, hyperactivity, and some incidence of disease as well as increase calcium absorption and reaction time to light.
- Use lighting as a way to play up interesting features and colors and draw the eye toward positive, mood-enhancing artwork or views.

Air Quality and Temperature

Indoor air pollution can pose many health risks and produce significant health effects (Desqueyroux, Pujet, Prosper, Squinazi, & Momas, 2002). Ambient air pollutants can cause a variety of respiratory problems, including bronchitis, emphysema, and asthma. Acute respiratory obstructive diseases such as asthma have been linked to smoking and to allergic reactions to dust mite feces, cats, cockroaches, and certain pollens (Dossey, Keegan, & Guzzetta, 2000; Evans & Kantrowitz, 2002). Indoor levels of pollutants may be higher than outdoor levels.

Healing environments provide good air quality to those who inhabit them. Since spirituality involves a connection to the environment, a healing environment supports spirituality by providing a comfortable, healthy place for individuals to live and work. Guidelines for improving air quality include the following (Leibrock, 2000; Neumann & Mensik, 1993):

- Open windows to improve ventilation.
- Clean air ducts regularly.
- Test for gas leaks on a regular basis.
- Maintain equipment and perform repairs in a timely manner.
- Use plants liberally and provide clients with access to outdoor areas (such as solariums, outdoor gardens, and roof gardens) whenever possible.
- Use air filters, ionizers, or ozone purifiers.
- Clean carpets and upholstery regularly.
- Accelerate the off-gassing of new materials (such as fabrics, carpets, upholstery) by leaving the house, turning up the heat, closing the windows, and "cooking" the environment for 24 hours, then opening the windows to ventilate the environment.
- Prohibit smoking.
- Use aromatherapy.

Pleasant temperatures are important in a healthy environment. Both temperature and humidity can dramatically affect comfort levels and should be controllable by the individuals inhabiting the space. Blankets, blanket warmers, and fans can be provided in areas where body temperatures may fluctuate or in health care rooms that are normally kept cool (such as operating rooms, recovery rooms, intensive care units, or emergency rooms).

Smells

For centuries, herbal remedies have been used to heal. While the exact chemical compound responsible for the healing was not always known, the healing properties of plants are well-known and well-documented. Aromatherapy, a form of healing that uses the sense of smell to evoke feelings of health and well-being, is especially useful for mood elevation, pain control, and relaxation. For example, jasmine and rosemary increase beta waves in the brain and result in a more alert state, and lavender increases the brain's alpha waves, thus promoting relaxation (Fontaine et al., 2001).

Hospitals and health care clinics are well known for their often unpleasant odors or chemical smells. Since smell is acutely retained in memory (even more than sounds or visual images), strong-smelling cleaning agents should not be used near clients. Pleasant odors, flower arrangements, and plants can reduce stress, absorb odors, and help clean the air and are important components of any healing environment (Neumann & Mensik, 1993).

Noise

Noise is one of the most invasive aspects of most health care environments, and its reduction is one of the most important components of a healing environment (Wright & Sayre-Adams, 2000). But what is noise? Is it a particular sound? Is music noise? What about the sounds created by the tires of a car as it travels on the freeway? Is a ringing telephone or a beeping pager "noise"?

Noise is difficult to measure and its definition can be subjective. What is noise to one individual can be a welcome sound to another person. While other types of pollution are easier to quantify, noise pollution is difficult to define. It is transient so that when it stops, the environment is rid of it. There are differing opinions about how much noise pollution is too much.

Noise is measured in decibels, and sound levels in environments can vary widely. The "noise floor" is the level of continuous sound that characterizes a particular area. To be perceived, other noises must rise above this level. If the sound level is too quiet, conversations and unavoidable sounds then become distractions (Mazer, 2002).

Most individuals are not aware of the hazardous effects of noise. It is now known that the intensity and duration of exposure to ambient noise has been linked to hearing damage (Evans & Kantrowitz, 2002). In addition, noise can have the following effects (Bilchik, 2002; Carsia, 2002; Evans & Kantrowitz, 2002; Grumet, 1994; Hager, 2002; Leibrock, 2000; Petterson, 2000):

- It increases blood pressure.
- It alters the way the heart beats.
- It disturbs digestion and can cause upset stomach or ulcers.
- It increases the respiratory rate.
- It disturbs the function of the endocrine system.
- It can negatively impact a developing fetus.

- It may elevate neuroendocrine stress hormones.
- It delays healing.
- It increases pain perception.
- It may increase the need for medication.
- It increases stress-related conditions such as headaches.
- It disturbs sleep.
- It interferes with complex task performance.
- It can be a significant contributor to industrial accidents.
- It may lead to motivational deficits linked to learned helplessness.
- It intensifies the effects of drugs, alcohol, aging, and carbon monoxide.

Noise is one of the most noxious stimuli in most health care settings. Hospital noise contributes to the sleep deprivation, confusion, and disorientation of clients. In the health care setting, sources of noise may include equipment alarms, telephones, ventilators, and staff conversations (Fontaine et al., 2001). Studies have shown that noisy environments are less caring environments. The individuals working there tend to be less altruistic, less nurturing, and more disengaged with each other, and they tend to work with a restricted focus on single-minded agendas. They are more "burned out," suffer more from headaches, and possibly make more errors in diagnoses and/or treatment (Grumet, 1994). One study that investigated the noise levels common in hospitals found that the ambient noise level was equal to the volume of a jackhammer (Bilchik, 2002).

On the other hand, the relaxing sounds of running water and music can stimulate the production of endorphins, lower heart rates, and reduce the need for anesthesia (Leibrock, 2000). Yet many health care institutions have not incorporated this information into their environments. One recent survey found that only about 20% of hospitals had made significant changes to their environment (Bilchik, 2002). Many others have increasingly incorporated the "open office" (cubicle) design into their environment in an attempt to save money. The result has been noisier offices, less productivity, and much more work-related stress (Carsia, 2002).

The following suggestions are ways to reduce noise levels and create a healthy, healing environment (Carsia, 2002; Grumet, 1994; Leibrock, 2000; Mazer, 2002; Neumann & Mensik, 1993; Petterson, 2000):

- Choose materials that decrease the generation of noise without sacrificing aesthetics.
- Use carpeting. It can reduce ambient noise by up to 70%, prevent the generation of surface noise, and reduce the levels of impact noise (such as that generated by footsteps on the floor).
- Utilize a wall of draperies, which can absorb nearly half the ambient noise in a space, or transparent barriers in areas where conflicting activities take place.
- Limit exposure to noise by keeping radios, televisions, paging systems, loudspeakers, slamming doors, and even footsteps in the hallway as quiet as possible. Even conversations from the nurses' station or staff lounge can be disruptive to an ailing individual and should be evaluated.
- Reduce or eliminate the use of overhead paging or intercom systems and replace them with vibrating pagers or vibrating cell phones.
- Design work and healing spaces to reduce noise. For example, long, rectangular rooms increase sound reflection while irregularly shaped recessed areas along walls and ceilings diffuse sound waves. Metallic equipment should have rubber or plastic bumpers.

- Be a responsible consumer and look for noise ratings when purchasing products.
- Have your hearing tested on an annual basis.
- Use sound-masking devices such as wind chimes, water, or music.
- Consider the careful placement of cubicles, restrooms, work areas, break rooms, and equipment rooms when designing work spaces.
- Wear hearing protectors when exposed to loud noises.
- Educate others about noise and take action before noise levels become disturbing or unhealthy. Encourage staff to speak quietly or display signage that requests others to contribute to a quiet, healing environment.

The Healing Power of Music

Music is a powerful spiritual healing tool that has been linked to medicine throughout history. In Greek mythology, Apollo was the god of music, and his son, Asclepius, was the god of healing and medicine. Music has been used during rites of initiation, during funeral ceremonies, and during harvest and feast days (Dossey et al., 2000).

It has also been suggested that listening to complex music can produce the "Mozart effect," a phrase coined by Alfred A. Tomatis when he alleged that children under 3 years of age had an increase in brain development when they listened to the music of Wolfgang Amadeus Mozart. Listening to complex music can serve as a type of mental exercise; facilitate the firing patterns of neurons in the cerebral cortex; and improve concentration, intuition, intelligence, and healing (Campbell, 2001).

The music used in a healing environment should be chosen carefully to account for individual preferences, responses, and cultural variations. Music without words is most effective in healing environments. (For a detailed discussion of music therapy, see Chapter 7.)

Furnishings

Furniture, accessories, art, and flowers help create a home-like atmosphere in the health care setting and can influence a client's outlook, contribute to comfort and a sense of safety, and increase orientation to an often unfamiliar environment. If health care takes place in the client's home, modifications can improve the individual's life and reduce injuries (Mitka, 2001). For example, universal design principles (such as having the bathroom, bedroom, and kitchen all on the first floor of the dwelling) and safety features (such as grab bars in bathtubs, tacked-down carpet, and deadbolt locks) promote independence, prevent harm, and promote health. All of these are important in a healing environment (Mitka, 2001).

Elements that contribute to a healing environment in a health care setting are often characterized as "home-like" and include the following (Dose, 2000; Leibrock, 2000; Long, 2001; Neumann & Mensik, 1993; Ulrich, 2002):

- Clocks and calendars (they can reduce the incidence of disorientation)
- Family photos and get well cards (they can prevent disorientation)
- Small groups of sturdy, comfortable chairs and recliners that offer neck and lumbar support and are easy to get into and out of

- Flexible, mobile seating that allows for comfortable overnight stays by guests
- Available telephones
- Break areas for visitors and caregivers
- Upholstery that is comfortable, visually appealing, and easy to maintain
- Art that is an integral part of the surroundings; contributes to the ambience of an environment; considers the needs and clinical conditions of the clients; and strengthens the link between the local community, staff, clients, and visitors
- Access to family and pets
- Home-like architectural details (such as bay windows, balconies, and porches)
- Easy access to bathrooms, and safe and efficient bathroom features (such as heated toilet seats, automatic flush levers, and an internal odor exhaust system)
- Safety features to prevent falls (such as grab bars, proper lighting, and nonslip floor mats)
- Refrigerators, couches, tables, and reading lamps that resemble home-like surroundings

Special equipment used in patient care areas are also part of the furnishings of a healing environment and should be selected to reduce the need to expend excess energy, encourage independence, and be safe and effective.

Art can provide a special link to healing. Art can help provide a level of human comfort in an otherwise sterile environment and reduce a client's stress level in the process (Lumsdon, 1992). Some health care environments use patient-created artwork, murals, and canvases to soften an often cold, vast, interior hospital space. Hospital volunteers may also create paintings for patient care areas (Lumsdon, 1992).

Other considerations should be factored into the decision when deciding about the placement of art in a health care environment. According to Ridenour (2001), art installed in critical care areas should be chosen so that it does not impair the staff's ability to assess patient skin color. Yellow-toned artwork may make patients nauseous, and "hard-edged" abstract work may cause agitation. Burn units should use soothing, cool colors rather than hot or warm colors. Elder patients benefit from comforting images, while images of healthy children are not recommended in critical care units with sick children. Large amounts of red or orange in artwork can agitate patients and be associated with blood or trauma but may work well in areas where depressed patients are being treated. Finally, art should be chosen because of its quality and not because it matches the furniture or décor in the institution.

Wayfinding

Wayfinding refers to what people see, what they think about, and what they do to find their way from one place to another in complex buildings. According to Carpman (1991, p. 24), wayfinding involves the following five "deceptively simple factors":

1. Knowing where you are.
2. Knowing your destination.
3. Knowing (and following) the best route to your destination.
4. Recognizing your destination upon arrival.
5. Finding your way back.

Carpman (1991) also describes the many elements involved in wayfinding:
Site and building layouts, circulation systems (corridors, stairs, elevators, and escalators), interior/exterior signs, sign terminology, directories, floor- and room-numbering systems, previsit information, handheld maps, 'You-are-here' maps, emergency exit information, interior 'landmarks' (such as artwork or unique design features), color-coded areas (or floor lines or carpet), staff-training programs, wayfinding system maintenance. (p. 24)

Wayfinding should eliminate anxiety, yet it is a major problem in most large, complex buildings. Many public facilities, including hospitals, airports, office buildings, and zoos, are maze-like buildings that confuse and frustrate users who waste an inordinate amount of time and energy trying to find their way around and through the facility (Carpman, 1991). The average visitor or client must navigate 6 to 20 buildings in a typical medical center (Ridenour, 2000).

Carpman (1991) lists several reasons for wayfinding difficulties:

- Poor facility design
- Incremental institutional growth
- Disorganized informational systems
- Lack of understanding by the facility planner about wayfinding and its importance

Wayfinding is an important component of a healing health care environment, since disorientation can result in increased fatigue; headaches; increased blood pressure; increased feelings of stress, frustration, and helplessness; or, in the most extreme situations, life-or-death consequences. Consider the ailing elderly patient with a walker who likes being punctual and is already late for an appointment as she searches the maze-like hallways of the hospital for the laboratory. Or consider the ambulance driver who is transporting a seriously ill person and cannot quickly find the emergency room entrance to the local hospital. In addition, staff members who are continually asked to provide directions to those who are lost are taken away from their official work duties, become less productive, and become more stressed. Spiritually healing environments are supportive and relatively free from stress. The use of universal, appropriate navigational tools and symbols prevents wayfinding confusion for the health care professional and the client and contributes to supportive, spiritually-relaxing environments (Carpman, Grant, & Simmons, 1990; Carpman, 1991; Leibrock, 2000).

Wayfinding can be improved by following simple guidelines (Carpman, 1991; Carpman et al., 1990; Leibrock, 2000; Ridenour, 2000):

- **Wayfinding must be a part of the building design process during every stage of design.** Every time the building is renovated or changed, or departments change their location or function, wayfinding needs to be reevaluated to assure that it is still effective.
- **Wayfinding must be considered with the first-time visitor in mind.** In many complex facilities, people who work there are often familiar with their routes to specific destinations, but new employees or first-time visitors must spend extra time and energy finding their way around a poorly designed building.
- **The form of a building provides the strongest wayfinding cue.** Limited numbers of corridors and the use of personal collections (such as artifacts, sculptures, photographs, or paintings) provide important orientation cues. Wall

hangings and pictorial symbols can create mood and add color as well as provide visual clues of location.

- **Unique patient room entrances can help a patient or family member locate a specific room from among a long corridor of rooms.** Unique floor tiles, room carpet that is a different color from the hallway carpet, or private patient mailboxes at the entrance of a room are just some ways this differentiation can be accomplished.
- **Atriums and galleries (instead of long corridors)** are effective wayfinding tools because of their often-distinctive designs.
- **Consistent lighting; floor stripes; and the use of colors, color coding, and patterns** can differentiate various sections of a health care environment.
- **A view of the sky and the ground** helps maintain circadian rhythms in patients and prevents hallucinations and disorientation.
- **Clocks and calendars can improve time orientation.** Writing the date and time on a whiteboard is also effective. It is not helpful to mark off the days on a calendar, however, as this can contribute to a patient's sense of loss of another day.
- **Signs should have only one symbol on them** (preferably an international symbol, understood by people of all languages). Type size should be large enough and there should be sufficient contrast between the text and the background of the sign so the information can be easily read. The signs should be placed in areas with sufficient lighting. Too many signs can result in "visual clutter" and add to wayfinding confusion, so their use should be carefully considered.
- **Signs that use tactile and audible cues** as well as visual cues are important to individuals with differences in vision, reading, and learning abilities.

THE HEALTH CARE PROVIDER AS A HEALING ENVIRONMENT

According to Dossey et al. (2000), health care providers can play an integral part in the client's healing journey, but this requires attention to the provider's own healing environment, both internally and externally. The presence of a health care provider can be one of the most powerful tools for healing in the client's environment. The "energy fields of the two interact and form a new pattern of inter-penetration, spirit within spirit" (Dossey et al., 2000, p. 45).

Healing is a process of being or becoming whole and requires the emergence of a process of connection, a "right relationship" between the health care provider and the client. This right relationship encourages true healing and the dynamic process of emergence into something new, rather than a simple return to prior states of being.

Respect, compassion, empathy, effective communication, appropriate clinical skills, and positive intent are essential elements in this process. Clients and their families may be undergoing a tremendously difficult ordeal. Yet, if care is delivered in a way that incorporates all the elements of a healing environment (including positive, supportive staff), the experience can be a healing one. Healing environments, with all of their elements, play a crucial role in this dynamic process.

SUMMARY

Leibrock (2000) writes, "The power of a healing environment comes from the little things, the design details that empower patients to take responsibility for their own health" (p. xv). Through their understanding of the environment's role in healing, health care providers can help create and support sacred spiritual spaces and healthy environments that maximize patient control; support the culture and history of clients; and emphasize wellness, prevention, and self-care.

KEY CONCEPTS

1. Health care providers have the power to create spiritually healing environments that allow clients to access their "inner healer"—that phenomenon of healing that transcends social, cultural, economic, time, and space barriers and promotes healing.
2. A healing environment is one in which individuals are supported and nurtured, in which they feel spiritually calm, and in which health and well-being are promoted. A healing environment is a vital part of maintaining a healthy lifestyle and is just as important as eating properly, exercising regularly, practicing proper health care, and having meaningful relationships and support systems.
3. The creation of a healing environment involves attention to specific design elements as well as cultural- and age-specific details.
4. Healing environments engage all five senses. They maximize choice and independence and include attention to specific design details such as color, nature, lighting, air quality and temperature, smells, noise, music, furnishings, and wayfinding.
5. Health care providers are an integral part of the client's healing journey. The energy and intent they bring to their relationship with the client is essential to this journey.

QUESTIONS FOR REFLECTION

1. Think about your workplace for a few minutes. Would you consider it to be a healing environment? If not, what are some areas that need to be changed?
2. While you may not be able to impact the physical environment of your workplace, remember that you are a part of that environment. Your presence in a room impacts the client—your sounds, smells, and visual images. Are you a healing environment? If not, what might you do to become one?

REFERENCES

Bilchik, G. S. (2002). A better place to heal. *Health Forum Journal, 45*(4), 10-15.

Campbell, D. (2001). *The Mozart effect.* New York: HarperCollins.

Carpman, J. R. (1991). Wayfinding in health care: Six common myths. *Health Facilities Management, 4*(5), 24, 26-28.

Carpman, J. R., Grant, M. A., & Simmons, D. A. (1990). Avoiding the hidden costs of ineffective wayfinding. *Health Facilities Management, 3*(4), 28, 30, 34-37.

Carsia, T. (2002). Designing workspaces for higher productivity. *Occupational Health & Safety, 71*(9), 192-195.

Desqueyroux, H., Pujet, J. C., Prosper, M., Squinazi, F., & Momas, I. (2002). Short-term effects of low-level air pollution on respiratory health of adults suffering from moderate to severe asthma. *Environmental Research Section A, 89*, 29-37.

Domrose, C. (2002). A family affair. *NurseWeek, 7*(7), 22-24.

Dose, L. E. (2000). The art of good management. *Nursing Standard, 15*(6), 18-19.

Dossey, B. M., Keegan, L., & Guzzetta, C. E. (2000). *Holistic nursing: A handbook for practice* (3rd ed.). Gaithersburg, MD: Aspen.

Evans, G. W., & Kantrowitz, E. (2002). Socioeconomic status and health: The potential role of environmental risk exposure. *Annual Review of Public Health, 23*, 303-331.

Fontaine, D. K., Briggs, L. P., & Pope-Smith, B. (2001). Designing humanistic critical care environments. *Critical Care Quarterly, 24*(3), 21-34.

Garber, K. (1999). Doctored design. *Hospital & Health Network, 73*(2), 26.

Gilhooley, M. J., & Rice, C. (2002). Grow with it: The role of plants in health care facilities. *Medical Group Management Association Connexion, 2*(17), 17-18.

Grumet, G. W. (1994). Noise hampers healing and curbs productivity. *Health Facilities Management, 7*(1), 22-25.

Hager, L. D. (2002). Didn't hear it coming: Noise and hearing in industrial accidents. *Occupational Health & Safety, 71*(9), 196-200.

Hansen, J. (2001). Light at night, shiftwork, and breast cancer risk. *Journal of the National Cancer Institute, 93*(20), 1513-1515.

Hasselkus, B. R. (2002). *The meaning of everyday occupation.* Thorofare, NJ: SLACK Incorporated.

Healing environments in surgical suites. (2002). *OR Manager, 18*(3), 14-16.

Higgins, M. E. (2002). Architectural design and Alzheimer's disease: Creating holistic living environment. *Arizona Geriatrics Society Journal, 7*(2), 10-24.

Leibrock, C. A. (2000). *Design details for health.* New York: John Wiley & Sons.

Long, R. (2001). Healing by design: Eight key considerations for building therapeutic environments. *Health Facilities Management, 14*(11), 20-22.

Lumsdon, K. (1992). Hospitals recognize link between art and healing. *Hospitals, 66*(19), 68, 70.

Marcus, C. C., & Barnes, M. (1995). *Gardens in healthcare facilities: Uses, therapeutic benefits, and design recommendations.* Martinez, CA: Center for Health Design.

Martineck, T. L. (2001). Facility profile. *Health Facilities Management, 14*(8), 16-18.

Mazer, S. E. (2002). Sound advice: Seven steps for abating hospital noise problems. *Health Facilities Management, 15*(5), 24-26.

McColl, S. L., & Veitch, J. A. (2001). Full-spectrum fluorescent lighting: A review of its effect on physiology and health. *Psychological Medicine, 21*, 949-964.

Mitka, M. (2001). Home modifications to make older lives easier. *JAMA, 286*(14), 1699-1700.

Neumann, T., & Mensik, K. (1993). *The healing power of design.* Innovator. (Available from Center for Nursing Innovation and Corporate Communications, St. Luke's Episcopal Hospital, 3720 Bertner Ave, Mail Code 4278, Houston, TX 77030).

Petterson, M. (2000). Reduced noise levels in ICU promote rest and healing. *Critical Care Nurse, 20*(5), 104.

Ridenour, A. (2000). Signs of the times. *Health Facilities Management, 13*(2), 41-42.

Ridenour, A. (2001). Art for health's sake: A step-by-step approach to developing a facility art program. *Health Facilities Management, 14*(9), 21-24.

Rose, V. (1993). Mother earth: American Indian beliefs and practices in childbearing. *Midwives Chronicle & Nursing Notes, 106*(1263), 104-107.

Schernhammer, E. S., Laden, F., Speizer, F. E., Willett, W. C., Hunter, D. J., Kawachi, I., et al. (2001). Rotating night shifts and risk of breast cancer in women participating in the nurses' health study. *Journal of the National Cancer Institute, 93*(20), 1563-1568.

Spalding, B. (2001). A quiet place: A healing environment. *Support for Learning, 16*(2), 69-73.

Stichler, J. E. (2001). Creating healing environments in critical care units. *Critical Care Nurse Quarterly, 24*(3), 1-20.

Ulrich, R. S. (2002). What do we know about healing environments? *OR Manager, 18*(3), 17-18.

Voelker, R. (2001). "Pebbles" cast ripples in health care design. *JAMA, 286*(14), 1701-1702.

Wallace-Guy, G. M., Kripke, D. F., Jean-Louis, G., Langer, R. D., Elliott, J. A., & Tuunainen, A. (2002). Evening light exposure: Implications for sleep and depression. *Journal of the American Geriatric Society, 50,* 738-739.

Weber, D. O. (1996). Life-enhancing design. *Healthcare Forum Journal, 39*(2), 39-49.

Wright, S. G., & Sayre-Adams, J. (2000). *Sacred space.* Edinburgh: Churchill Livingstone.

PART III

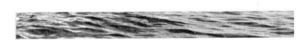

THE SPIRITUAL DIMENSION IN END-OF-LIFE CARE

Part III touches on the spiritual dimensions involved in caring for individuals at the end of life. This section examines:

- The spiritual care of the dying, including spiritual, psychological, and social dimensions
- Hospice and palliative care
- The advantages and disadvantages of dying at home
- Spirituality and the grieving process

9

SPIRITUAL CARE OF THE DYING

*"The most beautiful and most profound emotion we can experience is
the sensation of the mystical. It is the power of all true science."*
—Albert Einstein

LEARNING OBJECTIVES

Upon completing this chapter, you will be able to do the following:
1. Describe the spiritual, psychological, and social dimensions of dying.
2. Examine cultural considerations at the end of life.
3. List some interactions, caregiving strategies, and healing strategies that can assist health care providers in the spiritual care of the dying.
4. Describe the use of the senses in rituals for the dying.
5. Identify and describe aspects of hospice and palliative care.
6. List advantages and disadvantages of dying at home.

INTRODUCTION

What happens during death, that final life transition? With the knowledge of impending death, spiritual and religious beliefs play an essential role for individuals in making sense out of life. However, most people have done little to prepare psychologically, spiritually, or socially for death. Spiritual issues may not surface until individuals are faced with mortality. At that point, they often search for meaning in their own death or in the death of a loved one. Bereaved people may ponder the existential issues of life, not only with regard to the loss of a loved one, but for themselves as well as the life they once had. During this life transition, a person's most deeply held beliefs are challenged and opportunities for growth are experienced. To die peacefully and to die with the knowledge that life has had meaning is important to the dying person (Dossey, Keegan, & Guzzetta, 2000; Kuebler, Berry, & Heidrich, 2002; Lueckenotte, 2000).

In the past, health care has typically avoided the topic of spiritual care at the end of life and left clients to their own private beliefs and practices. However, as the interest in spirituality grows, care at the end of life is emerging as an essential dimension of holistic health care. Spiritual care is the work of all individuals involved in caring for the dying person. Spiritual care at the end of life means acknowledging and supporting the beliefs of the dying so that during the dying process, their needs are met (Flarey, 1999; O'Gorman, 2002).

Spiritual care of the dying considers and acknowledges the relationships of a person's life—relationships with the Ultimate, the self, and others. Spiritual care at the end of life provides an opportunity for the dying person to reflect on his or her successes, failures, hopes, fears, and sorrows. A framework for treatment decisions can be based on an understanding of the person's goals, values, and wishes, taking into account spiritual and religious as well as cultural beliefs (O'Gorman, 2002).

At the end of life, people usually go through a process of integration, an attempt to put the pieces of their life together in a pattern consistent with the whole of their life. This can include honoring significant relationships and commitments, exploring questions of meaning and purpose in life, engaging in relevant rituals, and making plans consistent with their values. Integration also involves the grieving and mourning of multiple losses associated with the ending of life. Spiritual integration is a healing process that provides closure and a sense of dignity as well as addressing unfinished business and mending broken relationships (O'Gorman, 2002).

Health care professionals can assist dying individuals and their families by incorporating the physiological, psychosocial, spiritual, and cultural aspects of dying into the care they provide and acting as guides to help the dying person and family members through this final life transition.

SPIRITUAL, PSYCHOLOGICAL, AND SOCIAL DIMENSIONS AT THE END OF LIFE

In addition to alleviating physical symptoms, care of the dying person should also meet spiritual, psychological, and social needs. The dying person is usually the best guide for what is best for him or her in this process. While choices may be made about the place of death (e.g., home, hospital, or hospice), the place of death is not as important as the care, trust, compassion, acceptance, and love that are provided and shared at this time (Dossey et al., 2000).

Spiritual Dimensions

Through transitions such as dying and death, an individual's most deeply held beliefs are challenged and opportunities for growth (or regression and despair) are presented. As Chandler (1999) writes, "Perhaps more than any other human experience, the hope of life after life, or even the fear of its absence, launches a spiritual journey" (p. 63).

Dying is a profound process of spiritual transformation. It is a spiritual event of enormous importance. Often, attention is turned away from the outer distractions in the world and turned inward, toward a greater peace and comfort in spiritual fulfillment.

To support individuals during this time of transition, the health care provider can help incorporate spiritual care into the plan of care. For example, if the hospitalized client is a practicing Buddhist with a fear of dying, providing quiet time and space for meditation could be a helpful intervention. If the person is a practicing Roman Catholic, experiencing the Sacraments might be essential to maintaining strength in the face of loss. If the person is a fundamental Christian, prayer and Bible quotations might speak to his or her soul. If the person is Jewish, providing foods that are appropriate to his or her traditions could perhaps give as much support as a half-hour of counseling (Collins, 2002).

If an individual is nonreligious, agnostic, or even atheist, discovering the central guiding principle for his or her life can be essential when providing quality care. Health care and spiritual care providers can use that knowledge to provide support and guidance. It is not important to agree with the beliefs or values, but it is important to recognize that a specific principle, reading, practice, or perspective is important and meaningful to that client. Since all persons are spiritual beings, it is only a matter of discovering what spirituality, life-perspective, self-transcendent resources make sense to the person receiving the care, and creatively and humbly using that perspective to bring healing and hope to the individual.

When family members struggle to assimilate and understand the dying process, they may find it helpful to seek as much information about the illness or condition of the dying person as possible. If they see the illness or condition as part of the person's life, they may find meaning in the person's life and in the illness or condition, be successful in maintaining family roles and relationships, address unfinished business, and advocate for appropriate treatment. The result of these tasks is a sense of peace and closure for the family (Burkhardt & Nagai-Jacobson, 2002; O'Gorman, 2002).

As part of the holistic process, health care and spiritual care providers should also come to terms with death as they assist families and clients in the dying process. The ability to respond to the many aspects of suffering creates a variety of situations for those providing spiritual care. For example, a provider's own experiences of death and dying, questions of meaning, and feelings of vulnerability may cause suffering as well. To further complicate the situation, the repeated attachment, detachment, and reattachment to new clients may be very distressing. Closure is a vital component of spiritual care for the provider as well as the client (O'Gorman, 2002).

Psychological Dimensions

In addition to spiritual considerations, a number of other factors are important in determining an individual's attitude and approach to impending death. One such factor is the psychological dimension. Psychological responses may be influenced by the client's age, sociocultural factors, religious background, physical status, level of social isolation or loneliness, and feelings about the meaningfulness of everyday life.

A variety of psychological symptoms such as anxiety, depression, sadness, and grief may be experienced at the end of life. Concentration may be difficult for the dying person due to physical symptoms or feelings of anxiety or depression.

Sadness can result from thinking about missing future events. The terminally ill may have worries about their families, loss of independence, pain, concerns about physical problems other than pain, and fears that they are a burden to their families.

In caring for the dying client, it is important for health care providers to anticipate these feelings, discuss them with clients and their families, and allay the client's fears and concerns. It is also important to anticipate the individual's need to grieve over the losses as death approaches (Kuebler et al., 2002; Lueckenotte, 2000).

Social Dimensions

Social needs at the end of life have to do with the individual's relationships and roles both within and outside the family, financial issues, and employment. Once the term dying is applied to an individual, role changes often occur. Social isolation often results as friends and sometimes family seemingly abandon the dying person. Not being able to work, not being able to drive, or not being able to participate in usual activities are dramatic changes that require adjustment. An attitude that people are ready to die and therefore have less need to interact with others fosters social isolation and may not be what the person desires.

During these transitions, clients may not express their feelings about the loss. Health care providers can assist clients through these transitions by acknowledging the losses, helping clients with their practical needs, and providing quality care at the end of life (Kuebler et al., 2002; Lueckenotte, 2000).

CULTURAL CONSIDERATIONS AT THE END OF LIFE

Customs pertaining to language, food habits, religious practices, kinship structures, music and movement, manner of dress, standards for modesty, reactions to fear, responses to pain, and so forth, are learned, shared and transmitted from one generation to another. (Ross, 1981, p. 4)

The cultural, ethnic, religious, spiritual, and social aspects of a society usually shape an individual's view of death and dying. Unlike ethnicity, which refers to an individual's membership in a group bound by common racial, religious, national, or linguistic backgrounds, culture refers to the learned behaviors, beliefs, and values that define an individual's experience. It affects the individual's views of health, illness, dying, and life after death. Because different cultures prescribe different ways of caring for the dying and rituals surrounding the time of death, culture may influence end-of-life care (Kuebler et al., 2002; Matzo et al., 2002).

Culture plays a prominent role and influences the decisions and behaviors of the individuals involved in the dying process. According to Ross (1981), culture does the following:

- Affects the assessment of comfort care needed for the dying and the kind of care provided.
- Influences the selection, perception, and evaluation of health care providers and their methods.
- Shapes beliefs about causes of death and dying.
- Determines preparation of the body and funeral and burial rituals and practices.

Cultural Competence

While the current cultural knowledge about death and dying needs further research, any effort to improve the quality of end-of-life care should be sensitive to cultural considerations, as one's culture provides a meaningful context for dying (Corr, Nabe, & Corr, 2003; Hallenbeck, 2001). Cultural competence and sensitivity on the part of health care providers helps individuals achieve a peaceful death within the context of their belief systems. Cultural competence addresses the many dimensions of culture, including ethnic identity, race, gender, age, differing abilities, sexual orientation, religion and spirituality, socioeconomic factors, and place of residency (Matzo et al., 2002).

Providing compassionate spiritual care means displaying sensitivity to all cultures and acknowledging the uniqueness of each individual. Because the information presented about the various cultures cannot be generalized to all people of a specific culture, it is imperative to ask the dying person and his or her family about specific beliefs, practices, and customs that may be important to his or her care while receiving treatment (Cobb & Robshaw, 1998).

Miscommunication among individuals of different cultures as they interact is caused by a lack of awareness of the various beliefs, communication styles, and decision-making approaches of the culture. However, an attitude of acceptance for all worldviews and belief systems helps health care and spiritual care providers avoid generalizations about any ethnic or cultural group and recognize that there are variances in all groups (Ekblad, Marttila, & Emilsson, 2000).

General Beliefs and Practices

It is essential to avoid stereotyping because no cultural group is a single, homogenous entity. For example, among Asian Americans, there are people who trace their ancestry to Cambodia, China, Japan, Korea, Vietnam, and other Pacific countries. A study that draws conclusions about blacks/African Americans living in New York City might not be equally valid for blacks/African Americans living in rural Alabama. Older Japanese Americans who were born in Japan may have very different views from the second generation born in the United States (Corr et al., 2003). However, the following section illustrates some general beliefs, practices, or customs related to several cultural groups.

- Some **Mexican Americans** believe that particular omens (such as the appearance of an owl or messages in dreams) are signs of an approaching death. Mexican American practices may include elaborate concern with death and the traditional religious celebration of the Day of the Dead (Lueckenotte, 2000; Ross, 1981). They may also include a unique form of grave art that is practiced during the Day of the Dead festival. Altars of food, flowers, pictures, candles, and artwork are placed on graves as a healing ritual for the living to come to terms with their loss, and therefore, make death less threatening (Luckmann, 1999; Wing, 1999).
- Some **Native Americans** believe in the concept of a "good" death or a "bad" death. A good death comes at the end of a full life and means that the person has prepared for death. A bad death is defined as a death that occurs unexpectedly and violently, leaving the deceased without a chance to say good-bye. Native Americans see the universe as a harmonious whole in which human

beings are one with nature. Death is a normal part of life, to be accepted like the changing seasons. For Navajos, care must be taken in handling the dead person's body or the spirit of that person may continue to threaten the members of the community in this world (Corr et al., 2003; Ross, 1981).

- In some **Asian cultures**, the loss of an older adult who is perceived as having accumulated years of wisdom and knowledge may be mourned more than the loss of an infant or a child. The child is viewed as having made a lesser contribution to society because of fewer years of life experiences. In the Chinese culture, the life-threatening aspects of an illness may not be told to the client. Instead, the client's family is given this information. When the client dies, the family often stays at the bedside. Clothing may be left at the hospital for a time to allow the "evil spirits" to leave. Some Chinese Americans tend to be stoic in the face of death, and death is a taboo subject among some Chinese Americans (Corr et al., 2003; Kuebler et al., 2002).

- In the **Jewish culture**, it is important to clarify who should be called as the client nears death. Any drains, catheters, or items that have the client's blood in them should be left attached to the body. The family may not want the hospital staff to touch the body because they may wish to perform a ritual washing after death. Some families may call a "burial committee" to make sure the body is prepared for burial according to Jewish law. Jewish religion dictates that burial should take place within 24 hours of death. Rather than taking the body directly to the morgue, special arrangements are often made for the body to be wrapped and taken directly to a funeral home. Traditional Judaism is opposed to embalming and cremation (Collins, 2002; Kuebler et al., 2002; Ross, 1981).

- For **Muslims**, death is considered a transition from one state of existence to the next state of existence, and they will reap the benefits of their endeavors on Earth in the life to come. Death is not considered a taboo subject for Muslims but rather an issue to be reflected on frequently. Muslims ideally wish to die at home. Many family and friends will come to be with the dying person, to pray for the person's welfare in this life and the life to come. If they practice Islam, members of the family will often remain at the person's bedside reciting from the Koran. When the person dies, the body should face in the direction of Mecca, the eyes and mouth should be closed, and the limbs should be straightened. The body is usually washed and shrouded in simple unsewn pieces of white cloth, a funeral prayer may be held in the local mosque, and a graveside funeral prayer may be said. Muslims prefer that the body be buried intact and as soon as possible (Ross, 1981; Sheikh, 1998).

Providing holistic, compassionate, spiritual care means that health care professionals understand the cultural differences that influence death and dying practices. Culturally competent care includes a commitment to respecting clients' and families' cultural values, beliefs, and practices.

SPIRITUAL CAREGIVING STRATEGIES

Health care providers can provide spiritual care of the dying by dealing with spiritual issues from the individuals' and the families' perspectives. One way to do this is to help the dying person achieve dignity in death. Another way is to listen to individuals who have a desire and a need to discuss their experience. Additional strategies, such as the following, can assist health care professionals to provide appropriate spiritual care of the dying (Flarey, 1999):

- Conduct a comprehensive assessment of the needs of the dying person and his or her family.
- Develop educational programs related to spiritual care and the growing trend of spiritual importance in the lives of individuals.
- Utilize a team approach to care, integrating clergy, social workers, and health care chaplains into the plans of care for the dying person.
- Obtain more education on strategies that adequately acknowledge spiritual experiences of the dying, regardless of your personal beliefs.
- Develop forums so health care providers can work through their own feelings regarding death and dying.

Interactions With a Dying Person

Dying is more than a medical event; it is a spiritual event. For all involved, it is a time for exchanging love, for reconciliation, and for transformation. The dying person's loved ones can become compassionate companions who help the dying person along this journey. Each person's death is as unique as his or her birth. People sometimes appear to "choose" their time of death, which is often influenced by the presence or absence of a family member or the passing of a significant date or time (Kuebler et al., 2002).

No one guide fits every situation, but the following suggestions may help family members and the dying person achieve a sense of peace during the final days of life (Corr et al., 2003):

- **Relate to the person:** Individuals and family members should relate to the person, not the illness. People who are dying need intimate, natural, and honest relationships. Hearing is the last sense to be lost, so be aware that dying individuals may hear all that is being said around them. This is often a good time to say good-bye and reassure them that the surviving friends and family will be "okay" and that it is "okay for them to let go." Saying these words may be helpful in assisting the person to have a peaceful death.
- **Be attentive:** Undivided attention is one of the greatest gifts anyone can offer to the dying person. Family members and health care providers can offer support by listening without judgment to the feelings and concerns of the dying person. By paying attention to nonverbal cues, they can discover specific needs, desires, and personal truths the dying person may be discovering. Laughing, listening in an interested way, and just silently being present are often appreciated.
- **Demonstrate compassion:** Placing a cool cloth on a perspiring brow; giving a backrub or gentle massage; holding the hand of a frightened, dying person; and listening to a lifetime of stories convey caring and acceptance of that individual.
- **Create a calm environment:** The human presence can be very healing, particularly in the final days of a dying person's life. Leaving room for silence and reducing distractions can create a calm and receptive environment for the dying person and his or her compassionate, healing care.

Healing Strategies

It is important to spend the final months, weeks, or days in a way that best suits the needs of the family, friends, and dying loved one. Music, art, dance, or poetry can give expression to the urge toward spiritual yearning and promote a peaceful environment. Some individuals may want to spend time talking or simply being together. Others might find it helpful and rewarding to engage in some of the following activities (Chandler, 1999; Corr et al.; 2003; Dossey et al., 2000; Kuebler et al., 2002; Roach & Nieto, 1997):

- **Journal writing:** Journal writing can be an extremely effective healing technique to use during the dying process. It can be done as a family or individual activity. As a family activity, family stories, recollections, and thoughts about the family's time together can be written down. Adding pressed flowers, photos, small mementos, and other items to a special book will help memorialize the life that is passing. For individual journal writing, the healing effect comes from the process of writing one's innermost thoughts and feelings.
- **Organizing family photos or a collection of favorite things:** Selecting photos to put in a special album and writing captions next to each photo can help younger family members enjoy family memories and appreciate their family's history. Organizing a collection of the dying person's special recipes, books, or other collectibles commemorates that individual's unique tastes and personality. Adding notes to any books also helps record memories about the person.
- **Planting a memory garden:** Planting a tree or memory garden is a living memorial to the dying person. As the plants grow, they will be a meaningful reminder of the loved one.
- **Enjoying pet companionship:** Depending on individual preference, AAT may bring comfort to the person who is dying. The dying person may also enjoy the company of a beloved pet and may even prefer this to visits from people who are not close friends or family.
- **Taking short trips:** If the person has the strength, going to a favorite place such as a park or favorite restaurant to enjoy some favorite foods may be therapeutic and can take the focus away from the illness. The person may be more interested in one last taste of a favorite dish than eating a carefully planned "prescribed" meal.
- **Using music to soothe the soul:** Music helps promote a client's physical, mental, and spiritual well-being. Music can be very beneficial at the end of life, when communications often break down and a sense of isolation sets in. Music may help the dying person achieve a deep state of relaxation, reduce pain and anxiety, improve mood, and uplift the individual's spirit. The key is to find music that will help the dying person feel a sense of relaxation and a sense of peace. Recordings of gentle environmental sounds such as ocean waves, wind, rain, birds, and music from harps, flutes, or stringed instruments may provide a sense of peace. However, not everyone likes music, so it is important to pay attention to the dying person's likes and dislikes.
- **Using art for expression of the spirit:** Art provides individuals with the ability to project their internal world into visual forms. Drawing, painting, or making a collage can be a way for the dying person to express his or her feelings about the end of life. For example, the dying person might draw his or her vision of the afterlife. The possibilities of using some form of art are numerous.

- **Engaging in spiritual reflection:** Many terminally ill people find it helpful to reflect on the spiritual aspects of life as they move closer to dying. Spiritual reflection involves asking some of the questions listed below.

Questions for Spiritual Reflection

- What have I learned about courage, strength, power, and faith?
- How am I handling my suffering?
- What will give me strength as I die?
- What am I grateful for?
- Am I involved in any spiritual or religious groups?
- Do I find meditation or prayer helpful?
- What do I need to do, or let go of, in order to be more peaceful?
- What provides meaning and purpose in my life?
- Do I have someone to turn to for communicating my thoughts and feelings?
- Do I have any unfulfilled goals?

The Use of the Senses in Rituals for the Dying

Touch, smell, taste, sight, and hearing are important senses in creating rituals for the dying person. A dying, bedridden person may be more sensitive to noise, perfume, cigarette smoke, and talking than many well-meaning visitors may realize. If the person is at home, he or she may prefer isolation (such as a bedroom), while others prefer to be where there is activity (such as in the living room). The following suggestions provide ideas on how the senses affect dying individuals, their caregivers, their family, and their friends (Dossey et al., 2000; Sulmasy, 1997):

- **Touch:** Touching is a powerful way to break the separateness, loneliness, and fear of dying. People who are dying may need touch more than ever. Touch can bring laughter, calmness, or tears. It can reduce feelings of isolation, reduce the symptoms of stress, and decrease pain and discomfort. Touch can bring healing to the dying, even though the disease is not curable. Simply sitting in silence and having their hand held may comfort dying individuals. However, due to some disease processes and treatments or particular cultural or personal beliefs, some people may find it uncomfortable and unpleasant to be touched.
- **Smell:** The sense of smell can elicit powerful emotions and evoke memories. For example, the smell of a rose may bring back memories of a special occasion and a special someone. Illness will probably change the types of fragrances that can be tolerated, and some odors may cause nausea or unpleasant feelings in the dying person. However, the dying person may be able to tolerate mild-smelling lotions and colognes. A long history of the use of aromatherapy and essential oils across cultures supports its effectiveness; the power of scent may help ease suffering and pain at the end of life in ways that are only beginning to be understood. Natural scents like rosemary or vanilla, a fragrant plant, or a mildly scented candle are best.
- **Taste:** The sense of taste varies for each individual and usually remains until the end of life. Sometimes a dying person's sense of taste is diminished and he

or she simply does not want to eat. When creating rituals for the dying person, provide foods that he or she desires. Tasting and eating have symbolic meanings for the person and the family. If the dying person no longer wishes to eat, this can be normal and does not cause undue suffering.

- **Sight:** Arrange objects that have meaning to the dying person within easy view. Visual items can include greeting cards, artwork, family pictures, or photos that have personal meaning. These objects should symbolize positive people, places, and events in the person's life. A room that has soft, subdued sunlight can provide a sense of serenity to surroundings. Light colors are usually more soothing to the dying person than bright or dark colors.
- **Hearing:** The sense of hearing is often sharp even to the end of life, so special words at death can be heard.

One way of helping individuals with spiritual tasks is to enhance opportunities for using their senses near the end of life. Providing opportunities for individuals to use their sense of touch, smell, taste, sight, and hearing can help them cope with dying.

The Moment of Death

Like birth, death is a natural stage of life. Preparing rituals for the moment of death is important, but overemphasizing the process could create a stressful environment that negatively impacts the dying experience.

To help the person achieve a peaceful crossing into death, health care providers and family members may touch, hold, talk, and be with the dying person in ways that deepen hope and faith (Dossey et al., 2000). Simply being present emotionally is a great gift that can be given to the dying person.

If healing rituals have been done prior to death, the dying person usually has a sense of serenity and inner calm. Before the person's eyes finally close, tight brow muscles may become relaxed and a sense of peace may appear on the face. Health care providers should continue to communicate with family caregivers and others who are there to support the dying person. They may shut the half-closed eyes of the dying person, stroke and hug the physical body (if appropriate), and adjust the head on the pillow for the last time. Depending on the dying person's beliefs, caregivers or loved ones may give him or her permission to "leave" and to meet others who have died before.

A "Good Death"

Gladys was 89 years old, suffering from Alzheimer's disease, and dying. She had been a schoolteacher for 30 years, attended church every Sunday, and had never married. Her family and friends were gathered around her. Gladys had mostly spoken in inaudible murmurs during the last few months of her life. But that last day, the day she died, she spoke words as clear as crystal. She spoke to her grand-nephew and asked him to sit by her. The family stood by in disbelief. Gladys was talking! She said "I love you" to all of them. Suddenly, she looked up as though gazing directly at someone and said, "I'm ready." They asked her who she saw and she said, "I see Mama and Papa, Francis, Bill, Albert, and Sam" (all people who had died before her). She then took her last breath, and left her family quietly and peacefully.

The spiritual experience of Gladys' death was enlightening and comforting to her family. They found peace and comfort in the fact that her passage into another realm or plane of existence was a beautiful experience shared by all who loved her.

HOSPICE AND PALLIATIVE CARE

For many individuals, being confronted with a terminal illness may be the first time they have faced their spirituality and their own existence; examined life's meaning and purpose; reevaluated relationships with themselves, others, and their Higher Power; and faced their impending death (West, 1996). The hospice and palliative care movement has helped people come to terms with terminal illness, impending death, and the importance of spiritual issues and needs (Cobb & Robshaw, 1998). Hospice and palliative care provide a blend of physical and spiritual care for dying people and their families. A team of nurses, physicians, social workers, psychologists, and pastoral care professionals may be utilized to address various dimensions of care, including spiritual care (Kellehear, 2000).

Two models of end-of-life care have evolved in the United States: "traditional" hospice care under the Medicare Hospice Benefit and palliative care. Hospice and palliative care have similar characteristics as well as some that are unique to each (Kuebler et al., 2002). Hospice care includes the provision of palliative care, but palliative care is both a method of administering comfort care and, increasingly, an administered system of care offered most often by hospitals.

Hospice Care

Founded in Great Britain in 1967 by Dame Cicely Saunders, Saint Christopher's Hospice was the beginning of hospice and palliative care. In 1978, the National Hospice Organization, now the National Hospice and Palliative Care Organization, was created to promote the care of the terminally ill in the United States.

The main goal of hospice care is to provide comfort, relieve pain, and promote quality of life. Focusing on palliation and extensive support services when a cure is no longer the goal of care, hospice care is a unique model of care (Perron & Schonwetter, 2001). A team that includes nurses, physicians, social workers, a chaplain, nursing assistants, and volunteers provides support. Other team members are added as specific needs arise and may include speech, physical, respiratory, and music therapists.

With hospice care, attention to the spiritual dimension is essential and central to hospice ideology and practice (McGrath, 1997). Spiritual interventions support the client and family and help them come to terms with death and dying. These interventions include assessing the spiritual needs of dying individuals and their families, designing interventions that recognize and assist in meeting those spiritual needs, and supporting a sense of completeness and closure to the individual's life. While hospice personnel cannot hope for a cure for their clients, they can hope for healing—the achievement of spiritual unity that produces wholeness of being.

Enrollment in a hospice program is available through several systems (Luggen & Meiner, 2001):

- The client's primary care provider determines if the client meets the criteria for hospice services and submits a referral.
- The client has a terminal diagnosis with a prognosis of 6 months or less.
- The client and the family agree to a palliative plan of care.
- After 6 months, a re-evaluation is made to determine if the client still qualifies for continued hospice management of the symptoms of the disease process.

Palliative Care

Palliative, or comfort care, recognizes that death is a normal part of life. Clients and their families receive physical, emotional, practical, or spiritual care from the start of a serious or terminal illness until the individual's death (Walter, 2002). Palliative care can be provided to any client in any part of a hospital, doctor's office, or less often, in the home.

Palliative care grew out of the hospice care movement and extends beyond the traditional hospice philosophy to include a broader approach of services for the terminally ill. The World Health Organization (2003) defines palliative care as the following:

> Palliative care is an approach that improves the quality of life of patients and their families facing the problems associated with life-threatening illness, through the prevention and relief of suffering by means of early identification and impeccable assessment and treatment of pain and other problems, physical, psychosocial and spiritual. Palliative care:

- Provides relief from pain and other distressing symptoms
- Affirms life and regards dying as a normal process
- Intends neither to hasten nor postpone death
- Integrates the psychological and spiritual aspects of patient care
- Offers a support system to help patients live as actively as possible until death
- Offers a support system to help the family cope during the patient's illness and in their own bereavement
- Uses a team approach to address the needs of patients and their families, including bereavement counseling, if indicated
- Will enhance quality of life, and may also positively influence the course of illness
- Is applicable early in the course of illness, in conjunction with other therapies that are intended to prolong life, such as chemotherapy or radiation therapy
- Includes those investigations needed to better understand and manage distressing clinical complications

A multidisciplinary team of personnel that includes physicians, nurses, social workers, occupational therapists, physiotherapists, dietitians, psychologists, and chaplains and/or pastoral care workers delivers palliative care. Palliative care services for the seriously ill, their caregivers, families, and loved ones include the following (Kuebler et al., 2002):

- **Curative or life-prolonging treatments:** Palliative care clients can receive all the benefits of comfort care while continuing curative treatments for their condition.
- **Relief of physical suffering:** Palliative care professionals provide highly skilled symptom management for pain, anxiety, constipation, weakness, and many other kinds of discomfort. They also provide both the client and the family with help in dealing with side effects of therapies.
- **Attention to emotional and spiritual needs:** Attention to emotional and spiritual distress is important. Palliative care teams can provide help with non-physical pain through counseling and spiritual support.
- **Communication:** The palliative care team is made up of medical and nursing practitioners, social workers, clergy, pharmacists, and physical and occupa-

tional therapists. An interdisciplinary team can facilitate open and frank discussions between all the people involved with a client's illness and can help their clients identify goals for their dying process.

- **Guarantee of 24/7 access to help:** Palliative care teams ensure that clients and their families can reach someone quickly when they have questions. Communication is coordinated between doctors, home care nurses, pharmacists, the hospital, and nursing home staff. Palliative care teams can arrange at-home care after a hospital stay and can organize help with transportation, at-home equipment, medications, and day-to-day decision making.
- **Support for the bereaved family:** After the person dies, palliative care programs don't forget about the family. They make sure that support and counseling services are available to those who need them.

How Do Hospice and Palliative Care Differ?

While both types of care place an emphasis on meeting the spiritual, psychological, and physical (relief from pain) needs of the dying, hospice care and palliative care differ somewhat in the location of care, the timing of care, payment for services, and the types of treatment offered. Table 9-1 illustrates these differences.

ADVANTAGES AND DISADVANTAGES OF DYING AT HOME

An estimated 25% of individuals die at home (Cobb & Robshaw, 1998). For dying individuals and their families, the advantages of staying in the home may include the following:

- Individuals and their families are free to do what they wish because their routines and schedules can be altered as needed.
- Continuous support of family, friends, and pets is available.
- The ability to prepare meals makes it easier to serve what the individual likes.
- The stress of traveling to and from the hospital or hospice facility is eliminated.
- The unique beauty of familiar surroundings provides comfort to the dying person.
- The individual and the family experience feelings and emotions in a different way because of fewer interruptions.

The disadvantages of staying at home may include the following:

- There may be inadequate support for, or difficulty in coping with, care needs.
- There may be competing needs for care by small children, older adults, or other sick or disabled family members.

Someday, dying in one's home will be commonplace, with loved ones present as they were long ago. Dying will no longer be an event for which a person has to leave home (Cobb & Robshaw, 1998). Health care professionals will come to the home and provide spiritual and physical care, give the families respite, and alleviate the dying person's pain and discomfort.

Table 9-1

Differences Between Hospice and Palliative Care

	Hospice Care	*Palliative Care*
Location of Care	Hospice programs far outnumber palliative care programs. Once a referral to a hospice care program is made, a team of hospice care professionals usually administers care in the home. Less often, care is provided in a specially equipped hospice facility or, even more rarely, in a hospital	While palliative care can be administered in the home, it is most often provided in an institution such as a hospital, extended care facility, or nursing home
Timing of Care	To be eligible for most hospice programs and to receive insurance benefits, the recipient must usually be diagnosed as "terminally ill" or within approximately 6 months of death	There are no time-of-death restrictions in palliative care programs. Care can be administered at any time, at any stage of illness, whether the individual is terminal or not
Payment for Services	Insurance coverage for hospice care can vary. Many hospice programs are covered under Medicare, and some hospice programs are subsidized for the economically disadvantaged or for individuals not covered by their own insurance	Since palliative care is usually administered through a hospital or regular medical provider, insurance usually covers it
Types of Treatment Offered	Hospice programs focus on comfort care rather than on the aggressive treatment of disease for individuals with a life expectancy of 6 months or less. Hospice care usually requires that clients give up curative or life-prolonging treatments	Palliative care provides a compassionate, comprehensive team approach to care that focuses on quality of life for anyone dealing with a serious illness, at any time regardless of diagnosis, prognosis, or treatment. Life-prolonging therapies may be utilized

SUMMARY

The dying experience is unique for each individual. As knowledge of issues involved in death and dying increases and positive attitudes are promoted, the spiritual care and support for people who are dying will improve. For many individuals, death is not an end to life. It is simply a passage to another dimension, sometimes called heaven, the spiritual world, another plane of existence, or nirvana. Regardless of one's personal beliefs and practices, helping dying individuals through the transition that leads to the ultimate peaceful moment of death and allowing them to express their own spiritual beliefs and practices are the greatest gifts a health care provider can give—or receive.

KEY CONCEPTS

1. In addition to alleviating physical symptoms, holistic care of the dying person includes the spiritual, psychological, and social care of the person.
2. Culture plays an important role in an individual's view of death and in a health care and spiritual care provider's provision of care at the end of life.
3. Dying is more than a medical event; it is a spiritual event. For all involved, it is a time for exchanging love, for reconciliation, and for transformation.
4. Touch, smell, taste, sight, and hearing are important senses in creating meaningful rituals for the dying person.
5. The hospice and palliative care movement has helped people come to terms with their terminal illness, impending death, and the importance of spiritual issues and needs.

QUESTIONS FOR REFLECTION

1. In addition to the ones discussed in this chapter, can you think of any other healing strategies that may be helpful in caring for a dying person?
2. This chapter included some advantages and disadvantages of dying at home. Have you experienced the death of anyone who died in the home? If so, what advantages or disadvantages did you observe?

REFERENCES

Burkhardt, M. A., & Nagai-Jacobson, M. G. (2002). *Spirituality: Living our connectedness.* Albany, New York: Delmar Thomson Learning.

Chandler, E. (1999). Spirituality. *Hospice Journal, 14*(3/4), 63-74.

Cobb, M., & Robshaw, V. (1998). *The spiritual challenge of health care.* New York: Churchill Livingstone.

Collins, A. (2002). Nursing with dignity, part 1: Judaism. *Nursing Times, 98*(9), 33-35.

Corr, C. A., Nabe, C. M., & Corr, D. M. (2003). *Death and dying, life and living* (4th ed.). Belmont, CA: Thomson/Wadsworth.

Dossey, B. M., Keegan, L., & Guzzetta, C. E. (2000). *Holistic nursing: A handbook for practice* (3rd ed.). Gaithersburg, MD: Aspen.

Ekblad, S., Marttila, A., & Emilsson, M. (2000). Cultural challenges in end-of-life care: Reflections from focus groups' interviews with hospice staff in Stockholm. *Journal of Advanced Nursing, 31*(3), 623-630.

Flarey, D. L. (1999). Touched by an angel of light: Care at the end of life. *JONA's Healthcare Law, Ethics, and Regulation, 1*(3), 5-7.

Hallenbeck, J. L. (2001). Palliative care: Intercultural differences and communication at the end of life. *Primary Care: Clinics in Office Practice, 28*(2), 401-413.

Kellehear, A. (2000). Spirituality and palliative care: A model of needs. *Palliative Medicine, 14*(2), 149-155.

Kuebler, K. K., Berry, P. H., & Heidrich, D. E. (Eds.). (2002). *End of life care: Clinical practice guidelines.* New York: W. B. Saunders.

Luckmann, J. (1999). *Transcultural communication in nursing.* Albany, NY: Delmar Thomson Learning.

Lueckenotte, A. (2000). *Gerontologic nursing.* St. Louis, MO: Mosby.

Luggen, A. S., & Meiner, S. E. (2001). *NGNA core curriculum for gerontological nursing.* St. Louis, MO: Mosby.

Matzo, M. L., Sherman, D. W., Mazanec, P., Barber, M. A., Virani, R., & McLaughlin, M. M. (2002). Teaching cultural considerations at the end of life: End of life nursing education consortium program recommendations. *Journal of Continuing Education in Nursing, 33*(6), 270-278.

McGrath, P. (1997). Putting spirituality on the agenda: Hospice research findings on the "ignored" dimension. *Hospice Journal, 12*(4), 1-14.

O'Gorman, M. L. (2002). Spiritual care at the end of life. *Critical Care Nursing Clinics of North America, 14*(2), 171-176.

Perron, V., & Schonwetter, R. (2001). Palliative care. *Primary Care: Clinics in Office Practice, 28*(2), 427-440.

Roach, S. S., & Nieto, B. C. (1997). *Healing and the grief process.* Albany, New York: Delmar Thomson Learning.

Ross, H. M. (1981). Societal/cultural views regarding death and dying. *Topics in Clinical Nursing, 3*(3), 1-16.

Sheikh, A. (1998). Death and dying: A Muslim perspective. *Journal of the Royal Society of Medicine, 91*(3), 138-140.

Sulmasy, D. P. (1997). *The healer's calling: A spirituality for physicians and other health care professionals.* New York: Paulist Press.

Walter, R. (2002). Spirituality in palliative care: Opportunity or burden? *Palliative Medicine, 16*(2), 133-139.

West, R. (1996). Nursing the spirit. *Australian Nursing Journal, 4*(1), 34-36.

Wing, D. M. (1999). The aesthetics of caring: Where folk healers and nurse theorists converge. *Nursing Science Quarterly, 12*(3), 256-262.

World Health Organization. (2003). WHO definition of palliative care. Retrieved May 6, 2003, from www.who.int/cancer/palliative/definition/en.

10

Spirituality and the Grieving Process

"It's okay to be afraid of things you don't understand.
It's okay to feel anxious when things aren't working your way.
It's okay to feel lonely... even when you're with other people.
It's okay to feel unfulfilled because you know something is missing.
It's okay to think and worry and cry.
"It's okay to do whatever you have to do, but just remember, too...
That eventually you're going to adjust to changes life brings your way,
And you'll realize that it's okay to love again and laugh again.
And it's okay to get to the point where the life you live is
full and satisfying and good to you...
And it will be that way because you made it that way."
—Anonymous

Learning Objectives

Upon completing this chapter, you will be able to do the following:
1. Describe the grieving process.
2. Identify types of grief responses.
3. Describe the spiritual dimensions of grief.
4. Describe cultural differences in response to grief.
5. Identify the goals of grief counseling and the elements of healing.

INTRODUCTION

Loss and grief are part of the human experience and can result from many types of life transitions. Spirituality is an integral part of loss and the grieving experience because during these times individuals often raise questions that are spiritual in nature, such as, "Why did this happen to me?" "Why did God (Spirit, Allah) take my loved one?" and "Why has He forsaken me?"

Loss can precipitate a grief reaction that may incapacitate an individual, or the event may become a catalyst for personal growth. A healthy response to loss and death is achieved when an individual attains a balance between his or her physical, psychological, emotional, and spiritual self. Spiritual beliefs can help people make sense of their lives, and the spiritual support of others can assist them through the dying experience.

THE GRIEVING PROCESS

Grief is a tidal wave that overtakes you, smashes down upon you with unimaginable force, sweeps you up into its darkness, where you tumble and crash against unidentifiable surfaces only to be thrown out on an unknown beach, bruised, reshaped. (Ericsson, 1993, p. 7)

All people experience grief differently, depending on their inner resources, support systems, and relationships (Dossey, Keegan, & Guzzetta, 2000). Individuals deal with many emotions during the grieving process. They struggle with spiritual issues and concerns, such as examining the meaning of experience, readjusting to life without the person who has died, and adjusting to the reality of the death (Doka & Davidson, 2001).

What Is Grief?

According to Davidson and Doka (1999), grief is a reaction to loss and is experienced spiritually, behaviorally, physically, and cognitively. Dossey (1997) defines grief as a normal response to loss, characterized as dynamic, pervasive, and individual. Lueckenotte (2000) defines grief as the acute reaction to one's perception of loss, incorporating physical, psychological, social, and spiritual aspects.

Strong feelings of grief are associated with certain losses, including the following (Davidson & Doka, 1999; Dossey, 1997; Lueckenotte, 2000):

- Death of a partner
- Death of a parent, child, or sibling
- Death of a relative or close friend
- Serious illness of a loved one
- Relationship breakup or divorce

Subtle losses can also cause strong feelings of grief, even though those closest to the grieving individual may not know the extent of the emotions felt by that individual. Subtle losses can include the following:

- Loss of health through illness
- Loss of physical ability
- Death of a pet
- Move to a new home

- Change of job
- Loss of financial security
- Graduation from school
- Leaving home

Grief may also involve the loss of power over choice and the human experience of that loss. An example of this type of loss might include someone who suffers a paralyzing injury. Grieving involves the gradual reorganization of one's life in a way that makes sense given the changed situation. This requires a new way of living—one that includes physical outlets, emotional expressions, spiritual experiences, and intellectual challenges in new and unfamiliar territory.

Characteristics of Grief

Characteristics of grief include the following (Rando, 1988):
- It involves many changes over time.
- It is a natural reaction to all kinds of losses, not just death.
- It is based on the individual's unique perception of the loss.

Grief is experienced as an individual reaction to loss. However, the first 2 years after the loss are usually the most intense (Doka & Davidson, 2001). Low periods tend to be less frequent after 2 years, but even after 2 years, people may still experience a sense of grief when attending special events, listening to a song, or looking at pictures of the deceased. The length of the grieving period may depend on the relationship with the person who dies, the specific gender and culture of the individual who remains, the circumstances of the death, the individual's support system and inner resources, and the situation of the survivors. One thing is certain—it can take a long time to recover from a major loss, and grief does not follow a prescribed timetable (Doka & Davidson, 2001; Kuebler, Berry, & Heidrich, 2002).

TYPES OF GRIEF RESPONSES

There are several types of grief responses, characterized by their cause, duration, and effects.

Acute and Chronic Grief

Acute grief may last up to 6 weeks, with the individual experiencing somatic symptoms of distress that cycle throughout this time (Luggen & Meiner, 2001).

Chronic grief is prolonged grief, and the grieving person never seems to reach a satisfactory conclusion. The bereaved is usually aware of the continuing grief. Feelings of guilt, anger, hostility, or ambivalence need to be resolved before the individual can move forward through the grief process (Luggen & Meiner, 2001).

Anticipatory Grief

Anticipatory grief occurs when individuals anticipate the death of a loved one (or themselves) or a perceived loss before the actual loss occurs. This type of grief includes the processes of mourning, coping, and preparations for a potential loss that begin when the impending loss is obvious. It may be affected by the duration and character of the illness, by concurrent stressors (financial, social, physical, emotional, etc.), by periods of uncertainty and certainty, by interactions with health care professionals, and by support (or lack of it) from others (Lueckenotte, 2000).

Anticipatory grief is a reaction not only to the expected loss, but also to all losses encountered, including the following (Doka & Davidson, 2001):

- The past that was shared and can never be regained.
- The present losses that occur and are experienced as a decrease in or end of possibilities.
- The future losses of the death and related losses such as loneliness, loss of hope, security, and events that will not be shared.

Anticipatory grief may be experienced by all involved—including the dying person. There have been many studies about anticipatory grief, and the results have been mixed. Some studies have found that the ability to anticipate a loss results in an easier grief experience, while others found no relationship between a period of anticipatory grief and the intensity of the postgrief reactions. Anticipatory grief has been shown, however, to reduce early shock, confusion, and depression (Lueckenotte, 2000; Roach & Nieto, 1997).

Anticipatory grief is more than a prolonged grief response. It is composed of many factors that contribute to its complex nature. When the loss does not occur as anticipated, anger or hostility may replace this response because the individuals who experienced anticipatory grief may feel deprived of completing unfinished business with the dying person.

Disenfranchised Grief

Grief that is not recognized or validated by others is referred to as disenfranchised grief. Individuals with disenfranchised grief cannot openly express their grief, may have no social support systems, may have unresolved family discord, and may have hidden relationships that are not revealed. This type of grief may be caused by the following (Lueckenotte, 2000; Luggen & Meiner, 2001):

- A relationship that is not recognized by others (such as cohabitation or same-sex partnerships).
- A loss that is not recognized (such as the death of a pet).
- A griever who is not recognized (such as the very old adult who may have dementia).
- A death that is disenfranchising (such as sudden deaths, suicides, or deaths caused by drunk drivers).

NORMAL GRIEF RESPONSES

Grief occurs in phases that people can move in and out of during the grieving process. However, it is best not to think of grief strictly as a series of stages. Grief can be like a roller coaster, with many ups and downs. Sometimes an individual may be doing well and other times not so well (Doka & Davidson, 2001; Kuebler et al., 2002; Luggen & Meiner, 2001).

Psychological Responses

Sadness is a common reaction to grief. It is not always easy to distinguish between sadness, which is a normal part of the grief process, and a prolonged, intense depression, which is an abnormal response to loss (Corr, Nabe, & Corr, 2003; Lueckenotte, 2000).

In addition to sadness, common (and normal) psychological grief responses include guilt, anxiety, anger, denial, depression, helplessness, and loneliness. Shock and disbelief may be experienced immediately after the death of a loved one, and the bereaved person may express a lack of self-concern, a preoccupation with the deceased, and a yearning for his or her presence. A sudden or accidental death may exacerbate the reaction of shock. Denial may follow soon after the initial shock. Anger may be directed at the deceased for "leaving" and creating a sense of abandonment or it may be directed at God or a Higher Power. Some individuals may also direct anger at themselves for not being able to save the life of the loved one. Guilt may stem from the bereaved thinking he or she could have done more or done things differently or from feeling angry at God or the one who died (Corr et al., 2003).

Sometimes the grief experience includes feelings of relief, especially if prolonged suffering or a difficult relationship was involved (Lueckenotte, 2000; McBride, 2002). Grieving persons may also recall positive memories of the one they have lost or the event over which they lost control.

As the grief period progresses, individuals may finally begin to feel like they are going to be okay. They begin to look toward the future, begin doing things for themselves, begin reconstructing their lives, develop new interests, and once again begin to seek experiences for personal growth.

Physical Symptoms

The physical symptoms experienced by individuals during the grief process can vary depending on many factors, including the individual's coping skills, level of social support, physical health, and the nature of the loss.

Typical physical symptoms experienced during a grief response include the following (Lueckenotte, 2000; O'Toole, 1997):

- Tearfulness
- Crying
- Loss of appetite
- Lack of energy
- Apathy
- Sleep difficulties
- Change in communication patterns
- Hypersensitivity to noise
- Change in libido
- Inability to concentrate
- Hypersensitivity to people or events

Additional physical symptoms include tension, weight loss or gain, sighing, feeling like something is stuck in the throat, tightness in the chest or throat, heart palpitations, restlessness, shortness of breath, dry mouth, and dreams of the deceased (Lueckenotte, 2000; O'Toole, 1997).

Social Changes

Grief can also involve social difficulties, which may include problems with interpersonal relationships or difficulty functioning within a working environment. The nature of an individual's social responses to grief and loss are related to the type of loss experienced. For example, a widow or widower may experience a change in roles. He or she may have to learn new skills that were formerly handled by the deceased, or there may be a change in socialization patterns. New relationships, new ways of interacting, and new communication skills may need to be learned. Individuals experiencing loss from a traumatic event may mourn the loss of life as they knew it before the event. They may mourn their perceived loss of freedom or the loss of their former physical self (Corr et al., 2003).

Depending on the type of relationship, and the social roles within the relationship, social changes may or may not be significant. If a person has established patterns of independent interaction outside of the lost relationship, the adjustment to new social roles may occur more quickly. How individuals deal with the experience of loss is one of the most profound factors in their happiness or unhappiness. Spiritual resources are essential in guiding people through this transition (Fischer, 1998; Lueckenotte, 2000).

Spiritual Dimensions

Dealing with loss and grief is one of the great challenges of life. Loss and grief often lead individuals to consider the existential issues of life and examine their lost loved one's life as well as their own. Spiritual searching for a sense of meaning or the realization that their value framework is not adequate to cope with this loss may cause difficulties. The grieving individual may be angry with God or experience a crisis of faith. Spirituality and a belief in something greater than the self are crucial components in a positive healthy grieving process and are highly individualized (Corr et al., 2003; Lueckenotte, 2000; McBride, 2002).

Health care providers can be an important resource for education and support during the grieving process. Allowing individuals to grieve in their own personal way is an important part of care. Individuals in the early stages of spiritual development may need more external support and communication, while more spiritually developed individuals may use rituals, rites, and symbols for comfort. Individuals in the last stage of spiritual development believe in connectedness to humanity, the world, and the universe, and may not need as much external support (Doka & Davidson, 2001; Dossey et al., 2000).

CULTURAL DIFFERENCES IN RESPONSE TO GRIEF

While the deep sense of grief and sorrow in response to loss is almost universal, cultural expressions of grief may vary. Each culture has developed its own beliefs, mores, norms, standards, and restrictions regarding responses to grief (Luckmann, 1999). Communication technologies, global news broadcasts, and extensive migration are also creating an environment in which traditional customs are increasingly changing.

Within each cultural group, variations in values and beliefs influence an individual's grief response. Key factors may include the age and gender of the mourner; family customs, values, and traditions; funeral and mourning rituals; the individual's faith foundation, geographical region, educational background, economic status, and prior experiences with death and loss; and the historical background of the cultural group.

Providing culturally competent care means identifying and responding to the specific needs of each family (Corr et al., 2003; Leininger & McFarland, 2002). For example, tears, moaning, sighing, and screaming may be similar responses to grief in people throughout the world, but variations in culture play an important role in an individual's view of death.

For the health care and spiritual care provider, it may be difficult to anticipate the needs of specific cultural groups, so it is essential to understand what the individual finds helpful, rather than relying on any one cultural group's traditions or beliefs. It is important to acknowledge and respect the diversity that exists among the different cultures so that stereotyping is avoided. However, understanding some of the common or shared grief responses found in different cultures can be a good foundational or starting point for understanding individual differences. While it is not intended as a detailed explanation of all practices among all cultures, this section presents some of the commonalities found among the major cultural groups in the United States.

Asian Americans

Since Asian Americans encompass many diverse cultural groups, they may have many different grieving expressions. In general, though, Asian cultures tend to have a stoic response to pain and grief. Some Chinese Americans may not publicly express grief, but some may feel comfortable expressing their grief publicly. Japanese Americans may respond to grief with denial or the repression of emotions and are likely to display an attitude of careful control over communication when grieving.

Chinese Americans and the grieving process are usually influenced by the religions of Confucianism, Taoism, and Buddhism. However, many are Christians as well as believers in other religions. Traditionally, the Chinese have believed that it is bad luck to talk about death. As in other groups, it is best to simply ask about the grieving needs of the individual (Giger & Davidhizar, 1995).

In some Asian cultures, the loss of an older adult who is perceived as having accumulated years of wisdom and knowledge may be mourned more than the loss of an infant or a child. The child is viewed as being able to make a lesser contribution to society because of fewer years of life experiences (Corr et al., 2003).

Hispanic/Latin Americans

The term *Latino* identifies all different cultures of North, Central, and South America. The Latino concept of *respeto* (rules guiding social relationships) explains the hierarchy in some Latino families. In this concept, higher status is given to older (vs. younger), and male (vs. female) family members (Shaefer, 1998).

Some Latinos also value the concept of *personalismo* (warm, friendly, personal relationships) and have the expectation that individual health care providers will be present, provide information, offer condolences, and seek out the needs of the family.

Some Hispanics view death to be "God's will" and display open expressions of grief. Typically, crying is conducted openly to express the loss of their loved one. Religion and spirituality are very important to almost all Latinos. Hispanics rely heavily on spirituality to cope with the loss of their loved one and their faith in God to comfort them in their grieving process (Doka, 2000; Luckmann, 1999;

Lueckenotte, 2000). As part of their spiritual expression, the family generally continues a relationship with the deceased through prayer and visits to the gravesite (Shaefer, 1998).

Native Americans

Beliefs, traditions, and ceremonies differ widely among the indigenous people of America; thus, the term *Native American* does not adequately describe the unique culture of each of the approximately 500 tribes (Shaefer, 1998).

The Navajo are the largest tribe in the United States. Spirituality is woven into the Navajo's daily experience. The Navajo believe the spirits of the dead are able to take the shape of natural objects. For example, spirits may take the form of whirlwinds and lightning. Contact with these spirits or dreaming about a person who has died may result in a lack of hozho (spiritual balance) and sickness. Burial usually takes place on or before the fourth day after death and during that time, a special ceremony may be performed to keep the spirit of the dead from trapping the souls of the living (Plawecki, Sanchez, & Plawecki, 1994).

The Sioux refer to themselves either by that name or by the ancestral tribal name of Lakhota. The Lakhota (An Alliance of Friends) are the second largest group of Native Americans in the United States, and they believe that death is a part of the circle of life (Shaefer, 1998). They believe that when people or animals die, they enter a neutral spirit land. The Sioux choose burial over cremation because they believe the spirit of the dead person resides in the body and should not be disturbed. A wake lasts from one to three nights, with evening prayers or religious services. A religious gathering to remember a person's spirit is held a year after the death. During this ceremony, family and friends tell stories about the deceased, distribute the deceased person's possessions to people who have helped the family most in the year following the death, and exchange practical gifts such as clothing and tools (Shaefer, 1998).

Like some Mexican Americans, some Native Americans believe in omens. Among Native Americans, grief tends to be family oriented, with all members assuming roles in the grieving process. They may or may not express grief publicly.

Blacks/African Americans

There is no one way that blacks/African Americans grieve, since they are a group of people from diverse ethnic, religious, and cultural backgrounds. In general, however, the black/African American community has a strong sense of spirituality that helps them during the grieving process. Inquiring about individual beliefs, traditions, preferences, and desires and being open and responsive to the wishes of family members enables the health care provider to support the grieving individual or family member (Corr et al., 2003; Doka, 2000; Leininger & McFarland, 2002; Shaefer, 1998).

Muslim Americans

Coming from many different countries of the world, Muslims share one religion, Islam. While burial rites are generally the same in most countries, grief reactions may vary. Depending on their country of origin, some Muslims will appear stoic when grieving and some will weep openly. Death is looked upon as the crossing over to the next world and eternal life (Shaefer, 1998).

Transcultural Communication

To communicate effectively with individuals from diverse cultures, health care and spiritual care providers need to understand the cultural bases for why individuals react as they do to grief, dying, and death. They also need to understand the influence of culture on specific rituals such as funeral and burial practices. A lack of understanding and sensitivity may lead to poor communication, misinterpretation of symptoms, misdiagnoses, and failed interventions (Corr et al., 2003; Luckmann, 1999).

Effective transcultural communication helps facilitate planning and intervention strategies that can be used to support grieving families. When health care providers encounter a client or family from a different cultural background than their own, it may be useful to ask about practices related to death and dying to help avoid misunderstandings (Corr et al., 2003; Hallenbeck, 2001).

Health care and spiritual care providers can help grieving families by encouraging them to discuss their loss and express their feelings (such as anger, anxiety, guilt, and helplessness). Health care providers can also provide families adequate time to grieve, allow for cultural differences, and provide continuing support as necessary. It is important to respect differences between and within the various cultural groups (Luckmann, 1999).

COPING WITH GRIEF

Coping strategies are important in adapting to grief (Roach & Nieto, 1997). Each person finds his or her own sources of comfort through such actions as joining a support group, participating in activities such as journaling, or engaging in spiritual or religious activities. Experiencing grief can be very stressful, so it is important to eat well, sleep well, and engage in adequate exercise (Doka & Davidson, 2001).

According to Feinstein and Mayo (1990), regardless of the individual's cultural background, working through grief means talking about the associated feelings and emotions, planning for the next phase of life, and developing insight into the events that have occurred. This process cannot be rushed. Working through grief requires time to accept that death has occurred and to work through the accompanying feelings. Ultimately, the individual who goes through the grief process may experience a sort of transformation from profound sadness to a sense of comfort.

GRIEF COUNSELING AND ELEMENTS OF HEALING

A grief counselor helps individuals understand their reactions to grief, accept the reality of their loss, work through the pain of grief, and adjust to a new life without the deceased. Seeing a counselor is recommended when the expressions of grief are destructive to self or to others, or in situations where the grief makes it difficult for the bereaved to care for themselves, others, or to function in roles such as in a job.

Seeking professional assistance to come to terms with a loss and work through grief is a sign of strength, not a sign of weakness (Doka & Davidson, 2001; Kuebler et al., 2002).

The goals of grief counseling are as follows (Lueckenotte, 2000):

- Assist and support the bereaved person through the grief process.
- Facilitate some level of integration of the traumatic event, including the emotions, meanings, and feelings that have been associated with it.
- Help grieving people recognize that emotional and physical pain are normal and healthy responses to loss.
- Allow them to accomplish these tasks in their own unique way.

Preparing for a grief intervention session is important and includes reviewing a client's history, cultural background, and type of loss experienced so effective interventions may be developed. If the health care professional is uncertain about his or her ability to work with a particular client, it is important to discuss those concerns and ideas for counseling with a trusted and experienced adviser.

During the counseling session, grieving clients may be asked to examine their previous experiences with loss and see how they have coped with similar experiences in the past. The counselor can also ask clients to be aware of their physical body sensations because body awareness is an important sensation to cultivate during the grief process. Most people are more aware of the weather or the time of day than of the sensations in their own bodies as they relate to grief and loss. Body awareness is a useful first step in helping clients reduce their level and intensity of grief. Keeping a diary of daily sensations and emotions often helps the person become aware of the physical and emotional expressions of grief (Lueckenotte, 2000).

Grief counseling involves the following 10 basic principles (Corr et al., 2003; Kuebler et al., 2002; Lueckenotte, 2000):

1. Help the individual actualize the loss. Health care and spiritual care providers can offer details of the death to the family and help individuals understand puzzling situations. Survivors of a traumatic event may need to be encouraged to talk about the loss.
2. Help the survivor identify and express his or her feelings. Guilt, regret, anxiety, helplessness, and other feelings can be expressed in many ways, including journaling, rituals, or crying.
3. Assist the survivor in living without the deceased. Survivors should be advised to postpone major decisions that involve life changes and to use their support systems as needed.
4. Facilitate the survivor's emotional withdrawal from the deceased. This should be done delicately and with sensitivity.
5. Provide the survivor as much time as needed to grieve the loss.
6. Help the survivor understand normal grief responses.
7. Allow for individual survivor differences and understand the cultural and social implications of grief.
8. Provide continuing support for the bereaved, including support groups, family, and friends.
9. Evaluate the survivor's coping skills and identify healthy behaviors (such as support groups) and unhealthy behaviors (such as alcoholism).

10. Assess the survivor for pathological responses (such as serious depression) and make appropriate referrals.

Grieving individuals are often quite tired. Grief work is exhausting, both physically and emotionally. When the individual is ready, it is important to work on reestablishing a balanced mind, body, and spirit so he or she can begin to accept the situation and resume daily life. The use of touch, music, comeditation (meditating, chanting, or praying together), and preplanned rituals (such as prayer circles) are often very helpful (Dossey, 1997).

After a death or a loss, the grieving individual should be encouraged to remember important anniversaries and maintain important rituals. Unsaid messages can be written in a letter and then burned so the message is "sent out to the universe" (Dossey, 1997).

Other specific interventions that can be suggested or taught during counseling sessions include the following (Dossey et al., 2000):

- **The value of forgiveness:** Guilt, self-blame, and anxiety can lead to depression. They rob the person of energy needed to heal, they reduce the ability to cope effectively, and they take important time away from establishing new relationships and positive life goals.
- **The value of becoming peaceful:** Centering, meditation, and contemplative prayer, as well as the use of relaxation scripts, are extremely helpful.
- **Blending prayers and breathing techniques as a ritual for relaxation:** There is a direct relationship between breathing and thinking, and this practice can reduce tension, fear, and pain.
- **Using mantras or prayers:** Mantras (the repetition of a word or sound, either aloud or silently) and prayers (the unique and spontaneous communication with a Higher Power or God) decrease loneliness and affirm faith in a Higher Power.
- **Reminiscing and conducting a life review:** These activities can help grieving individuals integrate their past, present, and future and work toward achieving a sense of peace.

During the grief counseling experience, the health care or spiritual care provider may explore the subjective experiences and effects of the experience with the individual and the family to determine the effectiveness of any interventions. Care of an individual who has experienced loss is considered an art. The health care professional can be an invaluable source of comfort, strength, and healing. Healing occurs when the person is assuming control, engaging in identity structuring, and relinquishing roles no longer appropriate. Manifestations of healing may include physical healing, increased energy, sleep restoration, immune system restoration, forgiving, forgetting, searching for meaning, and finding hope (Burke & Walsh, 1997; Dossey et al., 2000).

SUMMARY

Grief has no timetable and is a natural part of the human experience. A healthy response to loss and death is achieved when an individual is able to attain a balance between his or her physical, psychological, emotional, and spiritual self. Counseling may be beneficial for those having difficulty in coping with their loss. In a multicultural society, both providers and clients have much to learn from each other.

KEY CONCEPTS

1. Individuals experience grief differently, depending on their inner resources, support, and relationships.
2. Dealing with loss and grief is one of the great spiritual challenges of life.
3. Grief is subjective and can have psychological, social, and spiritual responses.
4. Although cultural expressions of grief may vary, the deep sense of loss and sorrow is almost universal.
5. Types of grief reactions include acute, chronic, anticipatory, disenfranchised, and dysfunctional grief.

QUESTIONS FOR REFLECTION

1. Think back to a time when you observed a client, friend, or family member whose response to grief seemed unusual or inappropriate to you. Is it possible that the person's response was based on different religious or cultural beliefs than your own? How can your new awareness of different grief responses help you to provide more sensitive, compassionate care in the future?
2. Ramona is a 64-year-old woman whose husband died less than 6 months ago. She tells you, "We were married more than 40 years. I just don't see how I can go on without him." What would be an appropriate, compassionate, and sensitive response? How would your response be different if her husband died 5 years ago?

REFERENCES

Burke, M. M., & Walsh, M. B. (1997). *Gerontologic nursing: Wholistic care of the older adult.* New York: Mosby.

Corr, C. A., Nabe, C. M., & Corr, D. M. (2003). *Death and dying, life and living* (4th ed.). Belmont, CA: Thomson /Wadsworth.

Davidson, J. D., & Doka, K. J. (Eds.). (1999). *Living with grief: At work, at school, at worship.* Washington, DC: Hospice Foundation of America.

Doka, K. Y. (Ed.). (2000). *Living with grief: Loss in later life.* Washington, DC: Hospice Foundation of America.

Doka, K. Y., & Davidson, J. D. (Eds.). (2001). *Caregiving and loss.* Washington, DC: Hospice Foundation of America.

Dossey, B. M. (1997). *Core curriculum for holistic nursing.* Gaithersburg, MD: Aspen.

Dossey, B. M., Keegan, L., & Guzzetta, C. E. (2000). *Holistic nursing: A handbook for practice* (3rd ed.). Gaithersburg, MD: Aspen.

Ericsson, S. (1993). *Companion through the darkness.* New York: HarperCollins.

Feinstein, D., & Mayo, P. E. (1990). *Ritual for living and dying.* San Francisco: Harper San Francisco.

Fischer, K. (1998). *Winter grace: Spirituality and aging.* Nashville: Upper Room Books.

Giger, J. N., & Davidhizar, R. E. (1995). *Transcultural nursing: Assessment and intervention.* New York: Mosby.

Hallenbeck, J. L. (2001). Palliative care: Intercultural differences and communication at the end of life. *Primary Care: Clinics in Office Practice, 28*(2), 401-413.

Kuebler, K. K., Berry, P. H., & Heidrich, D. E. (Eds.). (2002). *End of life care: Clinical practice guidelines.* New York: W. B. Saunders.

Leininger, M., & McFarland, M. R. (2002). *Transcultural nursing*. New York: McGraw Hill.

Luckmann, J. (1999). *Transcultural communication in nursing*. Albany, NY: Delmar Thomson Learning.

Lueckenotte, A. (2000). *Gerontologic nursing*. St. Louis, MO: Mosby.

Luggen, A. S., & Meiner, S. E. (2001). *NGNA core curriculum for gerontological nursing*. St. Louis, MO: Mosby.

McBride, J. L. (2002). Spiritual component of patients who experience psychological trauma: Family physician intervention. *Journal of the American Board of Family Practice, 15*(2), 168-169.

O'Toole, M. T. (1997). *The Miller-Keane encyclopedia and dictionary of medicine, nursing, and allied health* (6th ed.). Philadelphia: W. B. Saunders.

Plawecki, H. M., Sanchez, T. R., & Plawecki, J. A. (1994). Cultural aspects of caring for Navajo Indian clients. *Journal of Holistic Nursing, 12*(3), 291-306.

Rando, T. A. (1988). *Grieving: How to go on living when someone you love dies*. Lexington, MA: D. C. Heath.

Roach, S. S., & Nieto, B. C. (1997). *Healing and the grief process*. New York: Delmar.

Shaefer, J. (1998). When an infant dies: Cross-cultural expressions of grieving and loss. Summary of a panel presentation at the Third National Conference of the National Fetal and Infant Mortality Review Program. Washington, DC: American College of Obstetricians and Gynecologists. Retrieved August 3, 2003, from www.acog.org.

PART IV

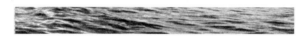

SPIRITUALITY
AND SPECIAL POPULATIONS

Part IV explores the spiritual considerations of special populations, including:
- Spirituality, religion, and children
- Spiritual dimensions of aging

11

SPIRITUALITY, RELIGION, AND CHILDREN

"This is my wish for you...
that the spirit of beauty may continually hover about you and fold you close within the
tendernesses of her wings... that each beautiful and gracious thing in life may be
unto you as a symbol of good for your soul's delight."
—Charles Livington Snell, in *This Is My Wish for You*

LEARNING OBJECTIVES

Upon completing this chapter, you will be able to do the following:
1. Describe the development of spirituality and religion in children.
2. Identify the relationship between the phases of psychosocial development and spiritual development in children according to Fowler, Piaget, and Erikson.
3. List the characteristics of spiritual distress in children.
4. Explain methods of providing spiritual care to children of various ages.
5. Describe specific care concerns for children with a chronic illness or for those who are dying.

INTRODUCTION

Proud new parents gently hold their infant as their priest pours water over the child's head. A congregation of friends and neighbors witness the baptism and welcome the infant into the Christian community. A Buddhist mother brings her child to a monk for consecration. On the eighth day after birth, a Jewish couple presents their son for his circumcision rite.

The acts described in the preceding paragraph represent specific rites of passage unique to a particular religious or faith community. While they often signify the beginning of a spiritual journey for the new family member, they do not guarantee that a child will follow that faith. In other words, as Carson (1989) writes, "Individuals may be born into a religious community but they are not born religious" (p. 25).

Just as the physical and emotional aspects of an individual need to be nurtured, the spiritual dimension of a person also needs care and "feeding." This care and nurturance often begins during infancy or early childhood (Betz, 1981). Elisabeth Kübler-Ross (1983) writes:

> ...all human beings are different, even before they were here. And then they are here to share this world with us, and all human beings have different lives, different experiences... Has anybody ever thought about the trillions of possibilities that life offers each one of us?" (pp. xii-xiii)

Through the support of family, friends, and a community of faith supporters, children are taught and guided as they travel on their own personal spiritual journey (Carson, 1989).

THE DEVELOPMENT OF SPIRITUALITY AND RELIGION IN CHILDREN

The development of personal spirituality is a dynamic, evolving process that occurs over a period of time. During this process, individuals become increasingly aware of the meaning, purpose, and values in their life. Faith, too, develops over time; it is an outgrowth of and a prerequisite for spiritual growth (Fulton & Moore, 1995).

An individual's spiritual development can be horizontal or vertical. Horizontal development involves the individual's relationships with the self, with others, with the environment or nature, or with spiritual activities. Vertical development involves transcendence and the individual's relationship with a higher power (Carson, 1989; Fulton & Moore, 1995). Children, too, develop their spirituality in both a vertical and horizontal manner. Their relationship with their parents or a caregiver begins both their vertical and horizontal spiritual journey.

Children may or may not come from a religious or spiritual background. Those whose families possess a strong religious background may not question who God is or what He does, while those without a strong religious background may learn about spirituality through their world experiences (Fulton & Moore, 1995).

Spiritual integrity is a basic human need, since it provides every individual's life with meaning. It influences values, relationships, and how people lead their lives. Spirituality in children is no different. Hart and Schneider (1997) state that spirituality in children is "the ability of a child through relationships with others to derive personal value and empowerment" (p. 263). Children's relationships with others as well as their relationships with a supreme being or values lead to the development of that spirituality.

Religious development, a component of spiritual development, involves the individual's "acceptance of a particular system of beliefs, values, rules for conduct, and rituals" (Carson, 1989, p. 26). Religious development may occur along paths similar to that of spiritual development or it may not.

Children, unlike adults, do not make clear distinctions between spirituality and religion. Yet, even very young children may have clear, often fluid, ideas about faith, prayer, and divine experiences (Barnes, Plotnikoff, Fox, & Pendleton, 2000). Shelly (1982) states that "stories abound of very young children who made serious and lasting commitments to God" (p. 12).

Religious and spiritual experiences can exert a powerful influence in the lives of children, influencing their moral development, their idea of social relationships, their way of perceiving themselves and their behavior, and their way of relating daily occurrences to a broader spiritual view (Barnes et al., 2000). A religious foundation in children has been associated with positive health-promoting and disease-preventing behaviors such as lower rates of adolescent pregnancy, suicide, delinquency, substance abuse, drinking, smoking, and violence. However, one potential negative effect of religious/spiritual involvement for a child is the risk of damage from a tradition that emphasizes guilt or the promotion of religiously sanctioned prejudice, hatred, or violence. In addition, a child may be considered at risk if the religion promotes a therapy that substitutes for medical treatment of an ill or injured child (Barnes et al., 2000).

While the cultural and spiritual convictions of a child and his or her family need to be honored, difficulties can arise for health care personnel when those convictions are at odds with the alternative forms of therapies perceived to be "better" for the child by mainstream medicine. A further problem may develop when the health care provider from a more traditional biomedical culture is not familiar with the child and/or the family's culturally based orientation and therapies and does not know how to relate to the family's viewpoint. This can result in pressure being applied to the child and/or the family to comply with the biomedical caregiver and a potentially dangerous impasse that can potentially harm the child (Barnes et al., 2000).

PHASES OF PSYCHOSOCIAL AND SPIRITUAL DEVELOPMENT

Many theorists describe the relationship between psychosocial development and the development of religion and spirituality throughout the various phases of life. This chapter examines the work of three theorists: Erik Erikson, a leader in the field of psychosocial development; Jean Piaget, a leader in developmental psychology; and James Fowler, who developed the stages of faith development and was greatly influenced by both Erikson and Piaget. (For additional information on Fowler's faith stages, please see Chapter 1.)

Please note that all three of these theories are based on Western experiences and a Judeo-Christian perspective. While this perspective may be the most familiar to many American health care providers, please see Chapters 4 and 5 to gain a broad insight into the role of various religions and cultures in the spiritual development of individuals from a wide range of backgrounds.

Infancy

While most people consider infants to be born without any defined spiritual self and without specific religious values, the time of infancy is a crucial one for developing faith, religious beliefs, and a personal spiritual dimension. This development is defined through the infant's experiences with his or her caregivers and lays the foundation for the infant's future spiritual beliefs (Carson, 1989).

- Erikson calls this period of psychosocial development (birth to 2 years) the stage of *trust versus mistrust*, when the foundation for hope and self-identity is established. At this stage, the infant's understanding of God is vague and the infant responds most to a warm and loving environment in which diversion, rather than punishment, is used to correct wrongdoing (Hart & Schneider, 1997; Hitchcock, Schubert, & Thomas, 1999; Shelly, 1982).
- Piaget refers to this phase (birth to 2 years) as the *sensorimotor phase*, since the infant primarily relies on its senses, motor skills, and reflexes to explore the world and solve problems (Hart & Schneider, 1997; Hitchcock et al., 1999).
- Fowler defines this stage of faith development (infancy to 3 years) as *stage 0* or *undifferentiated*, meaning that the infant does not have the ability to formulate ideas or communicate concepts about him- or herself or the environment (Betz, 1981). Infants have no sense of right or wrong and no religious or spiritual beliefs yet (Hart & Schneider, 1997). Their entire concept of self and the world is developed through the senses.

According to Shelly (1982), an individual's need for meaning and purpose is present from infancy. The need for love and connectedness is the foundation for survival. Babies who are unloved fail to thrive and may even die. When infants are cared for by a loving, kind, tender mother who meets their needs, they begin to develop trust and ultimately faith, which can be described as "a confidence or trust in a person or thing" (Betz, 1981, p. 22).

The infant's earliest spiritual need is one of unconditional love, and this need is initially met through the infant's relationship with his or her parents or primary caregiver (Hart & Schneider, 1997). Infants are completely dependent on their mothers (or primary caregivers) to meet their physical, emotional, and social needs, and these needs are met through touch and the senses. If their needs are met, infants develop a sense of trust. Through the process of trust, they begin to hope—hope that their needs will continue to be met in the future and hope that those closest to them will provide comfort. While the infant still has no concrete religious or spiritual beliefs (since they develop over time), trust and hope are the basis for the earliest development of both horizontal and vertical religious and spiritual development (Carson, 1989).

The development of trust is the foundation of a relationship with God because trust requires an openness and receptivity that are important characteristics of the relationship of an individual to a supreme being. If this foundation is not developed, individuals struggle with the ability to ever trust anyone other than themselves. Shame, doubt, and mistrust develop. If the foundations of trust, hope, and faith are developed, the infant possesses the basis for a relationship with God or an abstract being that is separate from self (Carson, 1989). The infant has a sense of belonging, self-worth, and a solid foundation for spiritual development. Parents are usually the individuals who engender this hope and trust. Thus, parents are primarily responsible for the spiritual care of their children (Shelly, 1982).

Toddlerhood

The time of toddlerhood is characterized as a time of independence and the mastery of skills as the toddler begins to take advantage of his or her newly developing motor skills. In terms of spiritual development, this time is an important one. The toddler gains a sense of self and self-worth through the mastery of skills such as toilet training. According to Hart and Schneider (1997), toddlers first experience faith as courage—often exemplified when they acquire a "will," defy authority (usually the parents), and say "No!" Autonomy and assertion are important characteristics in the development of faith and a spiritual identity.

- Erikson views this time (from 1 to 3 years of age) as one of *autonomy versus shame and doubt* (Hart & Schneider, 1997; Hitchcock et al., 1999) and characterizes it as a time during which the toddler struggles with issues of assertion versus acquiescence (Carson, 1989). The toddler needs love balanced with consistent discipline (Shelly, 1982).
- Piaget refers to this stage (age 2 to 4 years) as *preoperational thought and the preconceptual phase*, when the toddler is extremely self-oriented, sees things from his or her own point of view, and judges things based on their outcomes or consequences (such as punishment or obedience) to the self (Hart & Schneider, 1997; Hitchcock et al., 1999).
- Fowler does not have a specific stage of development for this phase of life.

Toddlers have difficulty conceptualizing a supreme being and do not have the ability to comprehend the significance of their own actions (Betz, 1981; Hart & Schneider, 1997). If there are no religious or spiritual beliefs in the family, toddlers will often create their own concept of a supreme being to explain the unexplainable.

Toddlers cannot make a distinction between what is real or what is supernatural. Stories that explain faith or spirituality need to be simple. The use of illustrations is particularly helpful in getting the toddler to understand spiritual or religious concepts. The toddler often believes that supernatural beings are magical. For example, they may envision God as an angel or a "friendly person" with whom they can communicate (Betz, 1981).

This stage lasts until the child enters school. If children do not develop a sense of self-worth, they may have difficulty recognizing the value of others. They may feel alienated, which can affect their ability to participate in religious or spiritual practices. If they do not feel loved, they may have difficulty believing that any other being (human or otherwise) could love them. This can influence both their horizontal and vertical spiritual development process. While the child at this stage does not think of this in logical, rational means, the perceptions created by this stage of development can result in misperceptions that persist throughout a lifetime (Carson, 1989).

Early Childhood

The school-aged child is often a physically rowdy youngster who is quite active and demands the attention of others. This child is becoming increasingly proficient in both language and motor skills.

- Erikson characterizes this stage as one of *initiative versus guilt* (ages 3 to 6 years) since the child wins approval and recognition by solving problems and finishing simple tasks (Hart & Schneider, 1997; Hitchcock et al., 1999).
- Piaget calls this the stage of *preoperational thought and the intuitive phase* (ages 4 to 7 years) (Hitchcock et al., 1999). The child is learning to think but is not yet able to think rationally or systematically. He or she is self-centered and thoughts are subjective. The child will often fixate on one aspect of an event and ignore others and is incapable of mentally reversing a series of events.

- Fowler calls this phase (ages 3 to 7 years) *stage 1* or the *intuitive-projective phase* (Hart & Schneider, 1997). During this time, faith development mirrors the form of the child's parents. The child is influenced by the actions of his or her parents, their religious behaviors (such as bowing their head in prayer), their experiences in church, as well as any religious stories and rituals that the family observes. Bedtime prayers, religious holidays, and mealtime blessings can have a profound influence on the child.

According to Shelly (1982), the child at this stage views God in terms of physical characteristics such as hair color, facial features, and clothing worn. The meaning of prayer is still vague, but rituals are important. The child understands simple Bible stories with clear singular themes. A conscience is beginning to emerge and the child fears punishment. As the child ages, the desire to please is strong and the child sees right and wrong as absolutes.

School-aged children begin establishing new relationships outside the family, and their peer group becomes increasingly important. The desire to conform is strong. At the same time, these children are becoming independent, more skillful and productive, and developing a stronger sense of their own identity (Fulton & Moore, 1995).

Children at this stage are attempting to learn how to balance what they want with what others want. The successful achievement of this task can impact horizontal and vertical spiritual development. Children at this age have a developing conscience and understand that God, or a Higher Power, is capable of rewarding or punishing specific behaviors. If children are taught that they are "bad" for disobeying strict rules, they may also view God as a strict "parent" who cannot possibly love them (Carson, 1989).

During this time, children may increasingly verbalize their perceptions of God to their family. Others may, in their own unique way, ask God for something special (Carson, 1989). They may see God in a magical way and try to manipulate him through specific prayers that ask for something in exchange for good deeds. In this light, they turn to God only when they need something and they never really internalize their love of God (Carson, 1989).

Middle Childhood

The child between the ages of 6 and 12 years is characterized as one who is trying to become proficient at doing things.

- Erikson calls this the stage of *industry versus inferiority* (ages 6 to 12 years). This child is concrete in his or her thinking and is beginning to develop some logical reasoning skills (Hitchcock et al., 1999). If children are successful in this stage of development, they can feel worthwhile about their self-image. This can translate into successful participation in spiritual or religious activities and the ability to relate to others in a meaningful way (Carson, 1989).
- Piaget calls this the stage of *concrete operations* and believes that children in this stage (ages 7 to 11 years) have concrete thinking processes but are developing the skills of inductive reasoning and beginning logic (Hitchcock et al., 1999). Young children begin to acknowledge that God or a Higher Power is indeed how their family and community have presented him. If children experience a belief that differs from what they have been taught, they often dismiss that belief as "wrong" (Betz, 1981).

- Fowler calls this phase (age 7 to 12 years) stage 2 or the *mythic-literal stage* and views it as one in which children are evolving in their understanding of what God "looks like." Some children see God as an angry parent, a "bogeyman," or a magical spirit in the sky.

Children at this stage are interested in understanding how God does what he does, since this is the age of skill mastery (Carson, 1989). They may be volatile or prejudicial in their behavior in an attempt to protect their belief systems from being challenged (Betz, 1981). Children at this stage may have a relationship with God that is based on the expectations of what God can, or cannot do, for them. For example, a child may state that God "answered my prayers by helping me in school" (Carson, 1989).

Explanations about faith and religion need to be concrete and visual for the preadolescent, although they can be more sophisticated than those for the school-aged child (Betz, 1981). These children are able to reason inductively and deal with concrete, observable items. They have difficulty with abstract thinking, but their ability to think is broadened by their interactions at school, which provides them with the opportunity to see other points of view and compare their ability to problem-solve and reason with other children (Ebmeier, Lough, Huth, & Autio, 1991).

Adolescence

Adolescence is a time characterized by rebellion against authority and conflict about previously held attitudes about personal values and beliefs. This is a time of great angst for most individuals.

- Erikson characterizes it as one of *identity versus role confusion* (Hart & Schneider, 1997; Hitchcock et al., 1999). This phase (ages 12 to 18 years) is characterized as a time of transition from childhood into adulthood. Adolescents begin to test their limitations, separate from their parents, and begin establishing their own unique self-image (including the clarification of their sexual identity). Peer relationships are very important and can influence their identity development. This is a time of intense conflicts that can center on who they are, what their life means, and what they hope to achieve in their life as an adult. Failure to achieve an identity results in confusion about who they truly are.
- Piaget refers to this phase as the *formal operations phase* during which abstract and deductive reasoning skills are developed (Hitchcock et al., 1999). Children must go through this process in order to develop a clear sense of who they are as individuals.
- Fowler calls this stage of faith development *stage 3* or the *synthetic-conventional stage*. Adolescents realize that they are capable of separating facts about God and their world from their previously imagined perceptions of what God was like. They become aware of spiritual disappointment. If their perception of God is different from the perception presented by those in authority (such as their parents), they may often accept the authority's perception. However, adolescents begin to question the standards set forth by their parents (Hart & Schneider, 1997).

This is a time of paradoxes. Adolescents reject parental values and norms because they do not want to conform to their parents' way of behaving. They want to experiment with peer group behaviors, yet the peer group also demands conformity.

Teens may adopt a carefree, hedonistic behavior pattern or may completely give in to the requirements of their social group. This is a time when some teens totally reject organized religion because of what it represents to their parents, while others may find that organized religion provides them with a much-needed peer group and the promise of comfort and happiness. Those adolescents who were raised in a household where there was no strong religious identity may seek out a religion that was rejected by their parents (Betz, 1981; Carson, 1989).

Adolescents seek answers to questions such as, "Who am I in relation to God?" and "How do I fit in the universe?" Teens can, at this stage in their spiritual development, begin to understand that they are unique individuals with infinite value, and this understanding can satisfy their need for recognition. Adolescents sometimes experiment with new personas to see which one best suits them as individuals. They may even present themselves differently in different situations and among different people (Carson, 1989).

If adolescents are hospitalized, they can experience extreme stress, intense psychological distress, and suffering. The intensity of their spiritual or religious needs often increases in proportion to the severity of the illness (Silber & Reilly, 1985). According to one study, most adolescents believe in God or a supreme being and almost half of those who were afflicted by a serious or fatal illness experienced a striking change in their spiritual concerns. The health care provider's sensitivity to spiritual concerns can be crucial in providing compassionate care to adolescents during such a difficult time (Silber & Reilly, 1985).

Table 11-1 summarizes the psychosocial, cognitive, and faith development stages described by Erikson, Piaget, and Fowler.

Spiritual Assessments of Children

As with an adult client, the spiritual care of a child begins with a spiritual assessment. The assessment of a child may require some modification from the examples presented in Chapter 6, depending on the child's age and developmental level. Broad, open-ended questions provide the most information about the child's beliefs and practices. For example, the child can be asked (Hart & Schneider, 1997) the following:

- Who do you talk to when you are in trouble (scared, lonely, or sad)? If the child answers, "My parents," ask who else they talk to at this time.
- What makes you feel better when you are scared (lonely, sad, etc)?
- What do you think dying is like?
- What does God (or insert a word they use in place of God) mean to you?
- What would you say to God (or insert a word they use in place of God) if you could talk face to face?

Children may often ask questions of the adults who are caring for them, including health care providers. They may "test the waters" to see how comfortable, honest, open, and nonjudgmental the adults are in discussing topics such as death. Children usually want short, succinct answers to their questions. One approach is to provide them with a minimal response and wait for another question. Another approach is to reflect back the question they ask and allow them to respond (Hart & Schneider, 1997). Listening to children, rather than talking at or down to them, will provide the most relevant information about their concerns and the most accurate pediatric spiritual assessment.

Table 11-1

A Comparison of Psychosocial, Cognitive, and Faith Development Stages

Stage	Erikson's Psychosocial Stages	Piaget's Cognitive Phases	Fowler's Faith Development Stages
Infancy	Trust vs. mistrust (birth to age 2): the foundation for hope and self-identity are established	Sensorimotor (birth to age 2): the child relies on its senses to explore the world and solve problems	Stage 0, undifferentiated (infancy to age 3): the child has no religious or spiritual beliefs yet
Toddlerhood	Autonomy vs. shame and doubt (ages 1 to 3): the child struggles with issues of assertion vs. acquiescence	Preoperational thought/preconceptual (ages 2 to 4): the child is extremely self-oriented	No specific phase
Early Childhood	Initiative vs. guilt (ages 3 to 6): the child wins approval by solving problems and finishing small tasks	Preoperational thought/intuitive (ages 4 to 7): the child is not yet thinking logically and has a self-centered and subjective view of the world	Stage 1, intuitive-projective (ages 3 to 7): a highly imaginative phase in which faith development mirrors the parents
Middle Childhood	Industry vs. inferiority (ages 6 to 12): the child begins to develop logical reasoning skills	Concrete operations (ages 7 to 11): the child has concrete thinking processes and is developing inductive reasoning and beginning logic	Stage 2, Mythic-literal (ages 7 to 12): the child is evolving in thinking; asks what does God "look like"
Adolescence	Identity vs. role confusion (ages 12 to 18): the child tests limits and begins to develop a unique identity and clarify life's goals and meaning	Formal operations (ages 11 to 15): abstract and deductive reasoning skills are developed	Stage 3, synthetic-conventional: adolescents can separate facts about God and their world from previously imagined perceptions

Depending on the child's age, a family assessment may also be necessary in order to obtain the most complete information about the child. This assessment can include many of the items presented in Chapter 6. In addition, observation of the family's behavior, including comments made by both the parent and the child, can be helpful. Noting the family's religious or spiritual preferences, observation of rituals and practices, and the use of religious or spiritual symbols can also provide valuable information about how to best support the child and the family during a time of spiritual distress. If the family's spiritual needs are addressed and supported, the child will be better able to handle the trauma of a hospitalization or serious illness (Hart & Schneider, 1997).

SPIRITUAL DISTRESS IN CHILDREN

Children, like adults, can experience spiritual distress. If the spiritual assessment results in a suspicion of spiritual distress, the following information may be useful in confirming the diagnosis and determining a plan of care for the child and the family.

Children may express a variety of behaviors indicative of spiritual distress, depending on their age and developmental level. School-age children, for example, may be angry, withdraw from interactions with other people, cry, or regress in their behaviors. They may have nightmares or be unable to sleep. Often these behaviors are observed at nighttime or at bedtime hours when they feel most vulnerable.

A summary of the most common types of behaviors observed in children with spiritual distress is presented below (Shelly, 1982):

- Bewilderment
- Anxiety
- A desire to undo, redo, or relive the past
- Crying
- Sleep disturbances
- Psychosomatic manifestations
- Depression
- Disturbing dreams
- Discontinued religious participation
- Self-destructive behavior
- Self-belittling
- Self-pity
- Fatigue
- Feelings of powerlessness
- Feelings of hopelessness
- Irritability
- Fear of being alone
- Feelings of uselessness
- Sense of abandonment
- Doubts about the compassion of a superior being
- Feelings of being spiritually empty
- Verbalizing that God seems very distant
- Verbalizing a desire to feel close to God

- Seeking spiritual assistance
- Displacing anger toward religious representatives
- Loss of affect
- Demanding behavior

Many members of the health care team can provide holistic care of the child in spiritual distress. For example, children may wish to talk to a spiritual care provider before they go to surgery; a child or family member may request a religious ritual such as a prayer or blessing before a particular procedure; or, if the client is an infant, the family may wish to have the child baptized or blessed before surgery or other procedures (Fina, 1995). The child or the family may ask for a quiet place for meditation or silent prayers or they may want to listen to music. They may also want to maintain spiritual rituals, such as bedtime or mealtime prayers, that provide them with a sense of constancy during times of stress.

PROVIDING SPIRITUAL CARE TO CHILDREN

When providing spiritual care to children, health care providers should make every effort to deliver it in a manner that is congruent with the child's developmental and psychosocial needs. Many children, because of their age or developmental stage, have limited ability to clearly and articularly communicate their needs and feelings in this area. Compassionate spiritual care should start with an understanding of the normal fears and concerns of children at their particular stage of development. Care should be presented in a way that the child can understand, and health care providers should be acutely sensitive to the child's evolving spiritual needs (Hart & Schneider, 1997).

In addition to these general guidelines for pediatric spiritual care, several specific recommendations for certain age groups follow.

Spiritual Care of Infants

When an infant is ill or hospitalized, spiritual care revolves around providing a normal, regular routine so the child's sense of trust is not disrupted. Consistent care, consistent caregivers, and parental involvement in that care are crucial. Emotional comfort and stimulation can be provided to the infant through activities such as holding, cuddling, talking to, and playing with the child.

The infant's parents need to be supported in their parenting skills and listened to when they express concerns about the child. If they believe that their child's illness is the result of some kind of punishment or that it is a religious omen, they may find it helpful to discuss their concerns with a spiritual leader or trained caregiver (Hart & Schneider, 1997).

According to Betz (1981), spiritual care of the parents of an infant can be provided by:

- Actively listening to their concerns and fears.
- Providing reassurance about their parenting skills.
- Supporting their religious and emotional support systems.

Spiritual Care of Children

In order to provide spiritual care to children, the health care professional should understand how they grow physically, socially, emotionally, and mentally. The spiritual needs of children vary according to their particular stage of development. For example, a nurse will soon discover that providing a 2-year-old with a detailed, clinical explanation of why he or she needs an injection is futile. The same is true about a child's spirituality. Health care providers often expect very young children to understand complex religious or spiritual concepts and then act perplexed when the children don't understand what is being discussed (Shelly, 1982).

The specific interventions that support the spiritual development of toddlers include helping them to focus on reality, relieving any feelings of guilt they have that their disease or condition is a punishment from God or a Higher Power, using their own support systems (such as parents) to help them understand that they are not "bad," and continuing the use of any regularly used religious or spiritual rituals such as bedtime or mealtime prayers (Betz, 1981). While many children believe that their illness, their parent or sibling's illness or death, or the injury or death of a friend is a form of punishment because they had "bad thoughts" or "did bad things," other children find comfort in their relationship with God or a Higher Power (Ebmeier et al., 1991; Kübler-Ross, 1983). The feelings they experience are often a result of their level of cognitive development.

Barnes et al. (2000) have suggested the following guidelines for health care practitioners interested in integrating spiritual and religious resources in the care of children:

- Know that there will be spiritual and/or religious concerns when caring for children.
- Understand your own spiritual history and perspectives and draw from that understanding when providing care.
- Become familiar with a variety of spiritual, religious, and cultural worldviews.
- Allow children and families to teach you about the specific practices integral to their perspectives.
- Develop relationships with a variety of spiritual and religious resources and individuals.
- Listen to clients and families as they express their spiritual needs or concerns.

SPIRITUAL CARE OF THE CHILD WITH A CHRONIC ILLNESS

Chronic illnesses often disrupt lives in many ways. A chronic illness experience can be one of the most stressful times in the life of a child and his or her family. The physical, social, emotional, and spiritual dimensions of a child can undergo alterations that often cause much despair.

Chronic illnesses are estimated to affect 7.5 million children in the United States each year. They can involve physical, physiological, and developmental states that can fluctuate from acute exacerbations to periods of stability during which individuals and family members collaboratively support one another in an effort to manage the condition (Fulton & Moore, 1995).

Children with chronic illnesses such as cancer are at a high risk for spiritual distress. They may experience depression, feelings of isolation, helplessness, inadequacy, guilt, and a variety of fears related to their changing body image. Weight loss, alopecia, loss of body parts, and the fear of a premature death are all experiences that can contribute to a spiritual crisis (Hart & Schneider, 1997).

According to Ebmeier et al. (1991), concern over body image is especially distressing during illnesses that occur in middle childhood or adolescence. For school-aged children, the most feared health care experiences include having surgery, receiving an injection, having a finger pricked for a lab test, being away from family, and worrying that someone else might "catch" their illness. Children experiencing chronic illnesses may not be able to develop or maintain relationships with their peers. They may compare themselves to their peers and focus on their differences or the changes that have occurred because of the illness. This can lead to intense feelings of inadequacy, leading to a loss of self-worth and hope. Ultimately, these feelings can greatly affect the child's ability to heal and can result in spiritual distress (Fulton & Moore, 1995).

Children with chronic illnesses who are hopeful, who believe they have a future, or who are optimistic or have a positive attitude or expectations may experience the ability to maintain, regain, or support their health condition. Spirituality and/or religious affiliations may provide a structure for these children so that positive coping strategies are developed. For example, spirituality can help children cope with the following types of issues (Barnes et al., 2000):

- Nighttime fear
- Hospitalization
- Cancer
- Terminal illness
- Death of a family member
- Racism
- Trauma
- Sexual abuse
- A sibling's illness or death
- Substance abuse
- Psychiatric problems

Spirituality provides children with the ability to hope, and this hopefulness helps them accept the limitations of their current illness or provides them with the ability to accept that they may be dying. While hopefulness in children and adolescents is similar in many ways to that of adults, adolescents, in particular, have expressed a greater intensity and range of hopefulness than adults (Hinds, 1988).

Fulton and Moore (1995) consider chronic conditions to be multidimensional experiences. Interventions should reflect the child's developmental level, the type of condition the child is experiencing, the child's coping strategies, and the family's unique psychosocial and economic variables. Holding, comforting, play therapy, adequate pain control, and allowing parents to participate in the child's care are examples of important interventions, since they support the child's and the family's spiritual life (Hart & Schneider, 1997). Other effective avenues of care include bibliotherapy (the use of poems, anecdotes, metaphors, storytelling, and journal writing) appropriate for the particular developmental stage of the child, as well as biographical scrapbooks and literature that the child finds meaningful. Finally, health care providers can use themselves as a powerful healing tool.

In caring for the child with chronic illness, health care providers should also be sensitive to the needs of the child's family. Siblings may experience many different outcomes as a result of their brother or sister having a chronic condition. They may develop higher levels of self-esteem as they help the family with responsibilities and activities around the home. They may develop greater empathy and maturity as they strive to cope with the impact of the chronic illness on their sibling. Conversely, siblings may also experience jealousy or resentment about the special attention the sick sibling receives. They may also experience sadness, loneliness, anxiety, or guilt if they feel they somehow contributed to the sibling's illness (Fulton & Moore, 1995).

Health care providers can help the various family members (including the siblings if their ages warrants it) to understand these feelings by educating them about the wide range of emotions that may be experienced. By their caring presence, health care providers can be a "safe place" for the child and family members to express their emotions and vent feelings that might be uncomfortable or unacceptable if they were expressed to other family members. Health care providers can provide counseling services (depending on their expertise and training) and they can also provide family members with spiritual care resources as well as community resources that may help the members cope with these emotions.

SPIRITUAL CARE OF THE DYING CHILD

In modern society, children are expected to outlive their parents. Yet according to the American Academy of Pediatrics (2000), approximately 53,000 children in the United States die each year from trauma, lethal congenital conditions, extreme prematurity, genetic disorders, or acquired illnesses. These causes are quite different from the causes of death in adults. However, the same basic components of compassionate spiritual care provided to adults should be provided to dying infants and children.

Holistic palliative care is concerned with the physical, psychosocial, and spiritual care of the child at every stage of the illness. This growing concern for the holistic palliative care of the dying child comes from studies showing that "many children with cancer experience substantial physical suffering in the last month of life and that, in the memory of their parents, attempts to control the child's symptoms are often unsuccessful" (Collins, 2002, p. 657).

Competent and compassionate care, including palliative care, places paramount importance on respecting the dignity of the child and the family. Health care providers need to support the family's and the child's expressions of disappointment, anger, grief, and suffering. Fears of abandonment and isolation are great, and the parents and child need reassurance that the health care team will continue to provide support and caring throughout the child's death and thereafter (American Academy of Pediatrics, 2000).

Spiritual support for the dying child and his or her family includes communicating with the child about death. This is often a taboo subject in many cultures, and many families as well as health care and spiritual care providers avoid it to avoid facing a frightening reality. However, many children are quite aware that they are dying, and open communication can reduce their feelings of isolation and anxiety (Collins, 2002). Kübler-Ross (1983) writes:

Every person, big or small, needs one person in which to confide. Children often choose the least expected person: a nurse's aide, a cleaning person, or at times a handicapped child who comes to visit them in a wheelchair... and since they have gone through the windstorms of life at an early age, they know things that others of their age would not comprehend... They become stronger in inner wisdom and intuitive knowledge. (p. 2)

Families and siblings need much support during the dying process and after the child's death. Survivor guilt, suicidal thoughts, inconsolable grief, withdrawal, and self-accusations are common and may require formal counseling, since the intense grief reactions may remain for at least 4 years. Siblings cope in a variety of ways depending on their developmental stage. Shock, anxiety, and resorting to familiar activities (such as play) are common (Collins, 2002). Siblings are also keenly aware of their parents' or family's pain and worries and cannot be fooled. If they are allowed to share in the sorrow, they can often provide support in the form of a hug, a smile, or an insightful comment. Sharing feelings with them makes the loss easier to bear and helps prevent them from feeling guilty or as though they are the cause of all the anxiety. Healthy children should be allowed to laugh, giggle, bring friends home, or watch television (Kübler-Ross, 1983).

Health care professionals often do not feel equipped to provide the type of care needed by dying children and their families. Lack of formal training, time constraints, lack of reimbursements for the time spent with the families, and the often extremely difficult emotional challenges of providing care are just some of the barriers to providing optimum holistic care (Wolfe, Friebert, & Hilden, 2002).

Providing a family-centered approach to the spiritual care of dying children and their families is an effective way to meet the special needs of these situations. Through the unique skills of a caring staff and a multidisciplinary team, the entire family unit can be supported and cared for during this most difficult time.

A Family-Centered Approach

Two little boys, Jason, age 4, and Matthew, age 6, were playing a game of ball in the street when a speeding car hit and severely injured Jason. Matthew ran into the house screaming that Jason had been hit, and his mother, who was inside the house at the time of the accident, called 911. Although Jason received immediate care at the scene and was rushed to the hospital, his injuries were too severe and he died several hours later. During his last moments, his family was allowed to be with him, touch him, and talk to him so that he "wasn't alone." While he was not fully conscious during this time, his family knew that he was aware of their presence as they prayed and held him one last time. The hospital staff asked his family about their spiritual and religious preferences and contacted their clergy to support them during their ordeal. Although grievous and distraught, they felt that Jason was loved and cared for during his time of greatest need.

SUMMARY

Spiritual integrity, whether it concerns children or adults, is a basic human need since it provides life with meaning. Spiritual development in children is dynamic and evolves over time, although some theorists have proposed that faith and spiritual development progress along a specific continuum of phases. Children, like adults, may experience spiritual distress, and the care provided depends on the child's developmental and psychosocial needs as well as family-centered issues. Through the unique skills of a caring staff and a multidisciplinary team, the entire family unit can be supported and cared for during this most difficult time.

KEY CONCEPTS

1. There are several theorists whose theories help explain the role of faith development in children; Erikson, Piaget, and Fowler are among the most well known.
2. The time of infancy is a crucial one in developing faith, a religious belief, and a spiritual dimension.
3. Toddlers have difficulty conceptualizing a supreme being, and they do not have the ability to comprehend the significance of what they are doing.
4. During early childhood, children view God or a Higher Power in terms of physical characteristics such as hair color, facial features, and clothing worn. A conscience is beginning to emerge and the child fears punishment.
5. During middle childhood, children have concrete thinking ability and are beginning to develop logical reasoning skills.
6. Adolescence is characterized by rebellion against authority and conflict about previously held attitudes about personal values and beliefs. Teens realize that they are capable of separating facts about God or a Higher Power and their world from their previously imagined perceptions, and they become aware of spiritual disappointment.
7. Children with chronic illnesses are at high risk for spiritual distress. Spirituality and/or religious affiliations may provide a structure for these children so that positive coping strategies are developed.
8. Support of the dying child includes support of the parents and siblings during the dying process and after the child's death.

QUESTIONS FOR REFLECTION

1. A health care provider's beliefs about a child's ability to understand spiritual matters can have a powerful impact on the type of care and communication provided. Take a few moments to examine your beliefs about children's abilities at various ages. What do you think a 5-year-old understands about death and dying? A 10-year-old? A 15-year-old? Do your beliefs coincide with the developmental phases presented in this chapter?
2. Sammy is an 8-year-old boy with terminal cancer. His family has decided not to tell him about his prognosis because they think he's too young to understand. One night during the night shift, Sammy tells you he knows he is dying and wants to talk about it. What do you do?

References

American Academy of Pediatrics. (2000). Palliative care for children. *Pediatrics, 106*(2), 351-357.

Barnes, L. L., Plotnikoff, G. A., Fox, K., & Pendleton, S. (2000). Spirituality, religion, and pediatrics: Intersecting worlds of healing. *Pediatrics, 106*(4), 899-908.

Betz, C. L. (1981). Faith development in children. *Pediatric Nursing, 7*(2), 22-25.

Carson, V. B. (1989). *Spiritual dimensions of nursing practice.* Philadelphia: W. B. Saunders.

Collins, J. J. (2002). Palliative care and the child with cancer. *Hematology/Oncology Clinics of North America, 16*(3), 657-670.

Ebmeier, C., Lough, M. A., Huth, M. M., & Autio, L. (1991). Hospitalized school-age children express ideas, feelings, and behaviors toward God. *Journal of Pediatric Nursing, 6*(5), 337-349.

Fina, D. K. (1995). The spiritual needs of pediatric patients and their families. *AORN Journal, 62*(4), 557-564.

Fulton, R. B., & Moore, C. M. (1995). Spiritual care of the school-age child with a chronic condition. *Journal of Pediatric Nursing, 10*(4), 224-231.

Hart, D., & Schneider, D. (1997). Spiritual care for children with cancer. *Seminars in Oncology Nursing, 13*(4), 263-270.

Hinds, P. S. (1988). Adolescent hopefulness in illness and health. *Advances in Nursing Science, 10*(3), 79-88.

Hitchcock, J. E., Schubert, P. E., & Thomas, S. A. (1999). *Community health nursing: Caring in action.* Albany, NY: Delmar Thomson Learning.

Kübler-Ross, E. (1983). *On children and death.* New York: Touchstone.

Shelly, J. A. (1982). *The spiritual needs of children.* Downers Grove, IL: InterVarsity Press.

Silber, T. J., & Reilly, M. (1985). Spiritual and religious concerns of the hospitalized adolescent. *Adolescence, 20*(77), 217-224.

Wolfe, J., Friebert, S., & Hilden, J. (2002). Caring for children with advanced cancer: Integrating palliative care. *Pediatric Clinics of North America, 49*(5), 1043-1062.

12

SPIRITUAL DIMENSIONS OF AGING

"Youth is a gift of nature, but age is a work of art."
—Garson Kanin

LEARNING OBJECTIVES

Upon completing this chapter, you will be able to do the following:
1. Describe the unique spiritual challenges of aging.
2. Describe the process of spiritual development in the aging individual.
3. Explain the relationship between loss, hope, spirituality, and aging.
4. Describe the relationship between love, sexuality, and spirituality in the older adult.
5. Explain the relationship between religion, spirituality, aging, and health.
6. Identify how spirituality and religion help the aging adult cope with personal difficulties, stress, surgery, chronic illness, and cancer.
7. Describe cultural wisdom and the role of spiritual elders.

INTRODUCTION

The second half of life is a turning point—a time in which personal, social, and cultural goals are quite different from those of the first half of life. Creating a new self-image, adjusting to physical and mental changes of aging, adapting to a simpler lifestyle, and seeking quality of life become important objectives that can be realized through the dynamic, integrative process of spirituality (McFadden & Gerl, 1990; O'Brien, 1999). A little more than 100 years ago, these goals were only dreams, since most human beings did not live long enough for issues related to the "second half" of life to be important.

As people live longer into old age, the human race is moving toward an unprecedented phenomenon. Only a century ago, the average life span was 45 years. Today, that life span has almost doubled (O'Brien, 1999). During the 1980s, age 40 was considered "over the hill" by many; today, more than 108,000 individuals in the United States are over 100 years old (Adler, 1995). By the year 2020, more than 52 million Americans will be aged 65 or older, and by 2030 almost one in five will be over 65 (Fischer, 1998). With an individual maximum life span that is now thought to be between 80 and 120 years of age, the "face of aging" is truly changing. The "third age" or "young old" now begins around age 75 to 80, and the "fourth age" or "old old" begins at age 80 to 85 (Baltes & Smith, 2003).

As longevity increases, society is becoming more and more concerned about issues such as extended life, ethics, and aging. People struggle with questions like, "Is it ethical to remove elders from their homes when they are no longer able to care for themselves?" or "Does a 95-year-old deserve the same medical interventions as a 45-year-old with a similar condition?" As life expectancy increases, there is a great deal of interest in what it means to live longer and age well.

Everyone ages, and nearly everyone has older siblings, friends, and parents, causing these issues to take on personal importance. Research has produced a greater understanding of the physical, emotional, economic, spiritual, and social aspects of this phase of life. For many, however, the concept of aging remains ambiguous. Is it an ascent or a decline? Despite the varied opinions about aging, one question remains: How can people continue to live longer and enjoy a life filled with meaning and joy?

THE UNIQUE SPIRITUAL CHALLENGES OF AGING

For many people in the United States, aging is viewed simply from a physiological perspective. Aging is depicted as a time of deterioration, a time when body systems "fall apart" and minds "weaken." Aging individuals often lose or deny their mind-body-spirit connection and do not want to be associated with their aging body, especially when a particular body part has lost is youthful capacity (Becker, 2002). Many Americans are deeply worried about living for many years in a nursing home once they become physically or mentally frail or suffer from a long-term illness (Koenig, 1999).

In addition to physical concerns, the aging process also involves spiritual concerns. Many older Americans believe that their spirituality is central to who they are as a person and that spirituality is a vital component of their entire well-being (Davenport, 2003). While many people talk about aging gracefully, "growing younger," or emphasizing the positive aspects of aging, others dwell on the losses and negative facets. Fischer (1998) addresses these apparent differences of opinion in *Winter Grace*: "The fact is that aging is both a descent and ascent... Aging is a paradox, the unity of apparent contractions... Emptiness can somehow be fullness, weakness can be strength, and dying can lead to new life" (p. 8).

Spiritual concerns in later life are often driven by these paradoxes. Enrichment can result from the achievement of many of life's major tasks—creating a family and watching one's children grow and become independent, achieving a career goal, paying off a mortgage, or succeeding in a personal, creative project. Yet, losses are also a part of the paradox. With the independence of children and freedom from responsibilities of child rearing comes the "empty nest." With an abundance of free time comes the loss of independence, friends, and partners. With the wisdom of age comes the depletion of energy or physical strength, regardless of the individual's luck or genes (Davenport, 2003).

Spirituality is a critical component of health and well-being for the aging individual and it becomes more important as a person grows older. A key element of that spirituality is a realistic perspective of what is involved in the aging process so the realities are neither over- nor undervalued.

A CHANGING PARADIGM

In the United States, late adulthood (the time from age 65 to death) is more prone to negative stereotyping than any other stage of life (Hitchcock, Schubert, & Thomas, 1999). This is due, in part, to the cultural emphasis on youth and beauty and anxieties about aging and death. Since the extension of life is a relatively "new" human experience, many aging individuals have no positive role models, and very few aging individuals have been provided with any real direction about how to deal effectively with end-of-life issues. Fewer still have a "road map" for their spiritual journey as they age.

Among most cultures, however, the aging journey is revered as a time of hope, a time of discovery, and a time of maturity that is to be embraced. Spirituality is encouraged and expected with aging. The aging Hindu Brahman, for example, is given special status and is expected to retreat from active family and social life so that he or she may "obtain spiritual self-realization through renunciation and contemplation" (Blazer, 1991, p. 61). Aging is seen as symbolic of the beginning of a new life task.

Here in America, only during the last few decades of the 20th century has an emphasis on spirituality shifted the focus of aging to include the dimension of life. According to Fischer (1998), rather than stereotyping the elderly, health care providers can view the later years as a time when diversity and true individuality can evolve. If this perspective is adopted, then every stage of life can be viewed as part of a journey toward that unique evolution as a spiritual human being. In the face of the paradoxes of aging, people can find amazing resources. Wisdom, reflection, strength, a sense of purpose, inner peace, and transcendence can result.

AGING AND THE HUMAN SPIRIT

According to Missinne (1990), human beings, as they age, have three fundamental needs. All three needs are equally important and interrelated in different forms and degrees. Each human being needs the following:

1. **Biophysical exchange:** The need to be in contact with the physical environment in order to live and to fully develop as a unique individual.
2. **Psychosocial exchange:** The need, through psychosocial contact with others, to develop and nourish our unique personality.
3. **Spiritual integration:** The need to "maintain and to illuminate ourselves beyond our existence" (p. 46).

For the older adult, spirituality can provide the following elements essential to a healthy life (Fischer, 1998):

- Spirituality promotes acceptance of the past, contributes to enjoyment of the present, and provides hope for the future.
- Spirituality meets a basic human need.
- Spirituality helps during stressful life events, increases an individual's understanding of the meaning of life, and helps in preparing for death.
- Spirituality provides support during phases of multiple losses and during the grieving process.

Benefits of Spirituality in Aging

The elderly population is highly spiritual and highly religious (Heintz, 2001; Isaia, Parker, & Murrow, 1999). Spirituality can provide comfort during times of loneliness or distress; bring relief from anxiety; and provide a sense of meaning, purpose, productivity, and self-integration. It can provide the older individual with the ability to adapt to a changing environment such as the shift from a familiar home environment to that of a hospital or long-term care facility. Spirituality provides a sense of self-esteem, and it is an important resource for coping with illness and in preparing for death (Fehring, Miller, & Shaw, 1997; Isaia et al., 1999; Levin, Taylor, & Chatters, 1994).

Even though physical functioning may decline as an individual ages, spiritual functioning does not necessarily decline with age. Isaia et al. (1999) report that there is "no evidence that the spirit succumbs to the aging process, even in the presence of debilitating illness" (p. 16). Spiritual awakening and development with aging can provide the individual with wonderful opportunities for growth and the release of old patterns and beliefs that are no longer relevant (Leetun, 1996). Faith provides the aging individual with the inner strength needed to transcend physical disabilities associated with aging and to develop the emotional resilience needed to achieve longevity (Koenig, 1999).

The aging process is an important step in an individual's spiritual journey and spiritual growth. Spiritual individuals strive to transcend the many changes as well as the losses that accompany aging and achieve a higher understanding of their life and meaning.

The Inner Journey of Aging

Aging involves an intense inner journey: an examination of life and accomplishments, relationships, challenges, dreams, and insights. Aging is a time of assessing and evaluating how one's life was lived and preparing for the end of life. Older people may be less distracted and freer to "think without boundaries" than at any other age. This can result in a significant breakthrough in the individual's ability to reach new spiritual heights (Seeber, 1990).

As the years pass, individuals often consider their physical and mental decline. This can lead to depression and spiritual despair, bitterness, negativity, and overdependence on others. For some, a serious or chronic illness, or the threat of death, can give their life transcendent meaning and help them view their lives from a larger perspective. For others, these life situations can challenge their spiritual beliefs and a spiritual crisis can result, leaving them to question their beliefs and their faith.

Faith can, however, provide individuals with a sense of meaning and a broader perspective from which to view their lives and relationships (Koenig, George, and Siegler, 1988).

SPIRITUAL DEVELOPMENT IN THE AGING INDIVIDUAL

Spiritual growth involves developing a sense of identity, creating and sustaining meaningful relationships with others and a higher being, appreciating the natural world, and developing an emerging realization of transcendence (McFadden & Gerl, 1990). Spiritual development starts early: "Beginning with the first cry at birth, the human psyche yearns for integration" (McFadden & Gerl, 1990, p. 35).

The spiritual goals of children, adolescents, and young adults are focused on acquiring skills and knowledge so they may become productive and fulfill their personal goals. The second half of life involves a different spiritual journey. Spirituality in the second half of life involves an ability to think abstractly, tolerate ambiguity and paradox, experience emotional flexibility, and commit to values that are more universal in nature (McFadden & Gerl, 1990). Not everyone, however, can achieve this state of integrity. Aging, alone, does not mean individuals can achieve integration with themselves, others, or the natural world, or achieve transcendence.

The developmental tasks of aging involve finding meaning and fulfillment in life and exploring the positive aspects of life. They also include the following (Hitchcock et al., 1999):

- Recognizing and accepting the limitations of self.
- Planning for safe living arrangements.
- Practicing healthy lifestyles.
- Continuing warm relationships with family and friends.
- Establishing affiliations with individuals in the same age group.
- Facing the inevitability of death and the death of loved ones.

Psychosocial development authority Erik Erikson refers to the developmental tasks of this stage of life as ego integrity versus despair. These tasks involve the integration of all the elements of the past and an acceptance that this is the only life to be lived. The goal of this time in life is to be able to look back on life as meaningful and fulfilling. The positive aspects of life need to be explored and individuals strive to review the contributions they have made to others and the world around them (Carson, 1989; Hitchcock et al., 1999). Facing one's own mortality is a major life task (O'Brien, 1999). If individuals fail to achieve these tasks, they face a sense of futility and hopelessness that they failed to accomplish what they wanted to in life. Anger, resentment, and feelings of inadequacy and worthlessness may result (Hitchcock et al., 1999).

James Fowler, who developed the stages of faith development, describes the stage of spiritual development of the older adult as one of universalizing faith (O'Brien, 1999). This phase represents the culmination of all the work of the previous faith stages and is manifested by a feeling of absolute love and justice toward all humanity. An individual in this stage of faith development is one who can "sacrifice himself or herself to meet the needs of others" (Berggren-Thomas & Griggs, 1995, p. 8). This stage of faith development is difficult to achieve and few people ever attain it. The individual who is truly at this stage of development answers to a higher authority than the world recognizes and is often seen as a subversive individual (Berggren-Thomas & Griggs, 1995). Health care providers should remember that chronological age may not fully indicate what stage of faith development an individual has achieved.

LOSS, HOPE, SPIRITUALITY, AND AGING

Loss in middle and old age can occur in many forms. It may include the loss of a spouse or partner, health, friends, a work identity, social relationships, a beloved pet, economic stability, or independence. Bereavement, the outward manifestation of loss, usually does not permanently affect the health of an individual, but it may cause many psychological symptoms. While some losses produce negative health consequences, some may result in positive changes. Increased support from family and friends, more social interactions, or the making of new contacts and the broadening of life interests may occur as a result of loss (Hitchcock et al., 1999).

Losses such as retirement, the death of a spouse, or a terminal illness can complicate the older adult's spiritual journey (Berggren-Thomas & Griggs, 1995). Death is one of the greatest spiritual challenges in the life of any person (Kremer, 2002). For aging individuals, an approaching death may create a need for forgiveness as well as an opportunity to review their life and acknowledge their accomplishments. Religious persons fear death less than nonreligious individuals, but they still may fear the dying process. Many older adults turn to spirituality and religion to cope with illness, the death of a loved one, or the anticipation of their own deaths. If dying individuals cannot reconcile their life and struggles or cannot ask for the forgiveness they need, they may experience a spiritual crisis (Berggren-Thomas & Griggs, 1995). Personal contact can help alleviate loneliness and provide an opportunity to address the issues of spiritual distress that may result from the losses of aging (Malcolm, 1987).

The Role of Transcendence in Aging

Spiritual well-being in the aging individual means confronting suffering, loss, forgiveness, and death. Not all individuals want to enjoy or participate in the opportunity to grow spiritually or become self-actualized, but many find spiritual meaning in these struggles. For those who do, feelings of harmony and connectedness can be achieved through self-transcendence. Ellermann and Reed (2001) define *self-transcendence* as "a person's capacity to expand self-boundaries intrapersonally, interpersonally, and transpersonally, to acquire a perspective that exceeds ordinary boundaries and limitations" (p. 699).

Gerotranscendence, the final stage in an evolution toward maturation and wisdom, is a form of transcendence unique to the aging individual. It is normally accompanied by an increase in life satisfaction and it involves characteristics such as a connection to earlier generations, little or no fear of death, an acceptance of the mystery of life, the discovery of hidden aspects of the self (both positive and negative), a shift from egotism to altruism, and a rediscovery of the child within (Wadensten & Carlsson, 2003).

Transcendence is an important predictor of mental health and well-being among middle-aged and older adults (Ellermann & Reed, 2001). Healing and hope are often the result (Leetun, 1996).

Hope, Spirituality, and Aging

Dossey, Keegan, and Guzzetta (2000) describe hope as "a desire accompanied by an expectation of fulfillment" (p. 98). It is future oriented, involves something the individual wants, and goes beyond merely wishing or believing. Hope involves envisioning the desired circumstances to become a reality (Burkhardt & Nagai-Jacobson, 2002; Carson, 1989). Hope is linked to trust and is strengthened by strong religious and moral values (O'Brien, 1999). Erikson describes it as the outcome of a balance between trust and mistrust and thus as the first developmental task of life (Carson, 1989).

Positive, healthy relationships with others and with a Higher Power provide the basis for hope. Without these connections, a sense of loneliness and isolation can lead to a spiritual crisis. According to Miller (1999), hope has two components: willpower, or will, and wayfulness. Willpower involves the desire to live, to survive, to recover, or to learn, while wayfulness refers to the object or person in which one hopes, or in which the person places his or her trust and confidence.

Hope is a vital element in healing, but hope is not the same as the promise of a cure. Having hope is also related to spiritual well-being (Burkhardt & Nagai-Jacobson, 2002). Spirituality and the faith it entails can provide the aging adult with a positive outlook on the particular life situation experienced. The aging person engaged in life struggles may, for example, hope for a resolution, hope for a closer relationship to a Higher Power, or hope for forgiveness. Spirituality and the intrapsychic strength of the aging individual can provide a source of help when coping with stressful life events. This can take the form of intrinsic religiosity (prayer, a sense of meaning and purpose, and transcendence) or extrinsic religiosity (social support) (Fehring et al., 1997).

Hope has a horizontal dimension (i.e., oriented toward earthly goals and relationships) and a vertical dimension (i.e., oriented toward eternal goals and relationships) (Carson, 1989). In Spanish, the verb for hope is *esperar*, which also means "to wait." This dual definition seems appropriate, since hope can involve the process of waiting for clarification about what is to come (Miller, 1999).

According to Miller (1999), research on the effects of hope and health have found that hope results in the following:

- A greater number of goals being set by an individual
- More difficult goals chosen
- More personal happiness
- Less distress
- Better coping skills when dealing with difficult life situations
- Faster recovery from physical illness and injury

Miller (1999) further states that one of the health care provider's first duties to a client is to inspire hope through the development of a therapeutic relationship and the provision of appropriate and accurate health education and information.

Closely tied to the loss and hope experienced by older adults are the spiritual needs of forgiveness and reminiscence. According to O'Brien (1999), the process of forgiving one's self and others, especially in the face of a serious or terminal illness, can be difficult and involve a long and complex process of healing. Reminiscing about past events can often give rise to the need to forgive. While it may be hard for the individual to let go of past transgressions, forgiveness can help elders reframe their self image and make peace with the past.

Love, Sexuality, Spirituality, and Aging

Love is personal, universal, and the source of all life. It prompts each person to live from the heart, it encourages each person to choose, it underlies compassion and courage, and its relationship to health and healing is unexplained and wonderful (Dossey et al., 2000).

Individuals love in many forms. Children love their parents and grandparents, their favorite toy, or a beloved pet. As they grow, they experience their first infatuation or love of another person and all the emotions that go along with that experience. As individuals age, certain aspects of love are unique to growing older. These aspects include a love of self, others, and a Higher Power that can only be experienced after the many "trials and tribulations" of a life journey have been experienced (Fischer, 1998).

For aging individuals who have lost friends, family, loved ones, or a life partner, loneliness and isolation are common. They may celebrate their birthdays without cards, presents, family, or friends. They may not have experienced touch in a long time (Strong, 1990). This has been due, for the most part, to society's portrayal of what it means to age. American culture often views the aging American as unattractive, asexual, slow, and nonproductive (Reed, 2002). Yet, as Kübler-Ross (1983) so eloquently states, "We need the touching until we die... Old people would be less likely to drift into senility if they could rock a needy child... tell them stories or build dreams together. The little hands would explore old wrinkles and find them interesting and lovable" (p. 71).

Without a love for others or a love for a Higher Being, spiritually would not exist. Sulmasy (1997) writes that "spirituality is a relationship of love" (p. 13). The love people have for others and for God or the Ultimate Being is a spiritual relationship. Fischer (1998) theorizes that human love "enables us to trust that God actually loves us; it embodies that love, making it visible and tangible in our lives" (p. 88). Seeber (1990) adds, "To love with the whole soul is to love with all of the elan vital or the life-force within" (p. 49). The agape experience is one characterized by spontaneous, altruistic love that is achieved when the self is shared with others with no thought of reward. It is rarely achieved but is considered a spiritual virtue (Strong, 1990). Lasting love, whether it be from others, from God, or from some transcendence, allows individuals to fully experience their own wholeness. True healing and new life are the result (Leetun, 1996). The following example illustrates this type of love and spiritual essence.

An Act of Love

Madeline is an 82-year-old widow whose 86-year-old husband recently died of cancer. During the last years of his life, Madeline took care of her husband. She spent many days in the hospital with him, dressed and bathed him, and helped with his care. She believes these acts demonstrate her caring and love for a man she was married to for over 50 years. While it was emotionally draining for her at times, Madeline believes she is blessed. She has three children, seven grandchildren, and two great-grandchildren. She knows that by taking care of her husband, she passed on God's love and support through her love and support of him.

Madeline is one example of how spirituality can be expressed in older age. She has been able to reflect back on her life and find the purpose behind her existence. By reflecting on the past and believing in the future, Madeline finds meaning in the present.

For many people, spirituality is also reflected in sexuality and the physical expressions of love. Sexuality embodies the physical and emotional intimacy shared between people (Reed, 2002). It is an important part of who people are as individuals and it impacts how they interact with others as well as how they view themselves. While it does involve the physical act of intercourse, sexuality also involves the full and deep interactions with and connections to another person and with the universe. Love and sexual expression are often part of the respect and honor one person shows for another. Spirituality is an extension of that love and can be demonstrated through the caring, honor, and devotion that one person has for another.

Many individuals erroneously assume that sexual desires diminish with age, so the physical and sexual needs of aging individuals are often overlooked. However, stereotypes about sexuality and aging are beginning to change. Most research now indicates that while older adults may experience normal, age-related changes in their sexual systems and responses, sexual patterns persist throughout the life span. Most people maintain sexual interest and activity well into advancing age (Fischer, 1998; Reed, 2002).

Many older adults report that sexuality results in a higher quality life and it provides love, passion, affection, self-esteem, and affirmation of who they are as individuals (Lueckenotte, 2000). The older adult sees sexuality as a deep form of communication, and its expression may be more fully developed in the older adult than in the younger individual. Slower paced and more intimate concerns of empathy, nurturance, and deep joy may replace the more performance-oriented patterns of youth (Fischer, 1998). Health care providers should remember that the norm for sexual behavior in younger individuals should not be used as the norm for sexual behavior in the older adult (Fischer, 1998).

Spirituality means acknowledging the uniqueness of an individual. If older individuals are confined to a long-term care facility, tied to a wheelchair, and taken to places they may not wish to go, is their spirituality being honored? What if they are told when they were going to eat, be bathed, or put to bed? What if a couple in a long-term care facility is never given any privacy to express their feelings for each other? Providing holistic care means honoring the spiritual, physical, emotional, psychological, and sexual dimensions of the individual.

RELIGION, SPIRITUALITY, AGING, AND HEALTH

Many individuals, especially older adults, express their spirituality through their religion and religious practices and behaviors. Religion and associated activities are common among older adults; 9 out of 10 older adults rate religion to be important in their lives and say that its importance increases with age (Ebersole & Hess, 1998; Hunsberger, 1985; Mull, Cox, & Sullivan, 1987). They rate religious groups as the third most important source of support to older adults, following families and the federal government (Blazer, 1991).

While a fair amount of study has shown that church attendance is a fairly standard example of religiosity in young individuals, the same cannot be held true of the aging adult. Environmental and personal resources as well as physical function and physical or social limitations of the aging person, such as changes in mobility, often affect church attendance. Thus, church attendance among aging adults may more accurately reflect physical health, activity level, and mobility than a level of religiosity. As individuals age, decreases in church attendance are often offset by increases in listening to religious programs on the radio or in private Bible reading (Ainlay & Smith, 1984).

Spirituality is an important dimension of well-being for the elderly. A fair amount of research defines the complex connections between religious and spiritual beliefs and practices and an individual's physical and psychological health:

- Religiousness, or an individual's belief in a supernatural being, has been linked to recovery from and positive coping with breast cancer (Mickley & Soeken, 1993).
- Men and women coping with cancer who viewed religiousness as a major force in their lives and attempted to live according to the tenets of their faith reported less anger and hostility and greater transcendent meaning related to the disease than those individuals who practiced religion as a means to achieve personal goals (Mickley & Soeken, 1993).
- Individuals with ambivalence about religion or a lack of strong beliefs were shown to have more headaches, loneliness, worry and anxiety, and other mental health symptoms (Mull et al., 1987).
- Women tend to be significantly more religious than men in both their activities and their attitudes. Since widowers are less likely to participate in religious activities than married men, it is hypothesized that women serve as the social contact and religious "link" for their husbands (Cobb & Robshaw, 1998; Isaia et al., 1999; Mull et al., 1987).
- As religiosity increased, so did the individual's sense of purpose in life (Berggren-Thomas & Griggs, 1995).
- Older adults, particularly women, who attend religious services at least once a week appear to live longer than those attending services less frequently (Koenig et al., 1999).
- Religiosity among aging adults has a positive relationship with happiness, well-being, adjustment to life situations, and life satisfaction (Hunsberger, 1985; Kahn, 1995; Markides, 1983; Mull et al., 1987; Young, 1993).
- Religious elders who were racial minorities, had less income, and had poorer housing reported the same level of well-being as their white counterparts; this was attributed to contact with church-related friends and involvement in church activities (Mull et al., 1987).

Religiosity may be too complex a concept to simply be measured by church attendance. Therefore, studies of aging adults that try to correlate health status with religiosity in aging adults (as measured simply by attendance at religious services) may not be accurate (Markides, 1983; Mull et al., 1987). While much research supports evidence of a positive relationship between religion and physical health (Ebersole & Hess, 1998), other research (Schmied & Jost, 1994) shows no direct correlation between attendance at religious services and better health. More research is needed to address religiosity and spirituality and not just simply attendance at religious services.

COPING STRATEGIES FOR DIFFICULT TIMES

As people age, their feelings of self-worth may diminish. What factor prevents older adults from experiencing these feelings when dealing with declining health or retirement?

Religion provides individuals, especially the elderly, with effective strategies for coping with personal difficulties and stress. Religious coping strategies include obtaining personal strength or support from God or a Higher Being, using prayer to help cope with difficulties and stress, and seeking the guidance of a Higher Being when making important decisions (Krause, 1998).

Attendance at religious services, prayer, Bible study, or listening to religious radio or television programs elicits "good feelings" and provides comfort to aging individuals. Prayer, in particular, provides the individual with a sense of power—to pray for friends in need, for health, and for strength during difficult times (Young, 1993).

Spirituality, Religion, and Surgery

Spirituality becomes very important for most older adults during the stress of hospitalization, health care procedures, or surgery. During this time, individuals reflect on suffering, death, and their relationships with self, others, and a Higher Power in order to make meaning of their life.

In addition, the most important and commonly used coping strategy in the acute care setting is prayer. Religious beliefs and practices have been linked to the survival rate among surgical patients.

Spirituality, Religion, and Chronic Disease

Due to rapid advances in health care technology, individuals can now live into old age with heart disease, Parkinson's disease, diabetes, multiple sclerosis, and other chronic diseases. As the burden of chronic illness grows, the importance of addressing how to care for individuals living with chronic illnesses also grows.

Clinical studies are beginning to clarify how spirituality and religion contribute to the coping strategies of many clients with severe, chronic, and terminal conditions (Post, Puchalski, & Larson, 2000). Chronic illness can lead to a renewed faith in or relationship with a Higher Power, or it can have a devastating impact on an individual's spiritual growth and sense of wholeness. Those with chronic illnesses often perceive themselves to be different from others, and they may experience intense feelings of loneliness. Chronic illness often signals the end of one way of life and a need to use a different set of skills to adapt to the changes presented by the illness (Young, 1993).

Healthy friends of the chronically ill person may withdraw because of their discomfort about the illness or their wish to minimize the discrepancy between themselves and the ill person. Chronically ill individuals may experience conflict about whether to suffer alone or share their fears and concerns with those closest to them. Individuals with neurological disorders such as stroke or Parkinson's disease often find their sense of isolation compounded by their inability to communicate with others in a socially acceptable manner (Miller, 1985). Loneliness can lead to a loss of self-esteem, negativity, depression, self-loathing, and spiritual distress or a spiritual crisis.

Spirituality may play an important part in the well-being of the chronically ill. It provides individuals with an ability to cope with their condition, thereby improving their physical and mental health. It can also counteract negative feelings and promote a feeling of productivity. Spirituality allows the person to "reconcile with the past, accept the present, maintain a positive view of life, and achieve life satisfaction" (Young, 1993).

Spirituality, Religion, and Cancer

Spirituality and religious beliefs are central to coping with cancer and helping individuals find a meaning in their having the disease. Older adults with cancer often experience guilt, fear, anxiety, and resentment. Having faith in a Higher Power often helps them reaffirm the value and meaning of their lives.

Health care and spiritual care professionals can play a major role in providing spiritual care to people with cancer. A multidisciplinary approach is usually the most effective. Although many institutions provide clergy visits, nurses—in particular—spend a great deal of time with their clients. Individuals should be cared for in a way that preserves their uniqueness and their religious or spiritual beliefs. Ministers, priests, or other religious advisers should be included in the client's health care program. Privacy should be afforded and respected so the client can discuss confidential matters (Lueckenotte, 2000).

Older adults may have personal items with them such as a Bible, a Koran, a crucifix, a religious medal, a prayer shawl, handkerchiefs, small bottles with oil, or other religious or spiritual items that should not be tampered with or thrown away. If the client wishes to meditate, privacy should be maintained.

If a health care provider is uncomfortable with providing spiritual care to a client, assistance from another care provider may be necessary. Addressing spiritual and religious beliefs is an integral dimension of survivorship (Lueckenotte, 2000).

SPIRITUAL INTERVENTIONS FOR THE AGING ADULT

As with every other age, interventions for the older individual should be specific to each client's spiritual needs. Organizations can help individuals find meaning in life and enhance their spirituality through the following methods (Ebersole & Hess, 1998):

- Provide gerontological education to clergy in seminaries as well as training to existing religious and health care staff.
- Develop outreach and visitation programs to homebound elderly.
- Create prayer circles.
- Provide telephone reassurance programs.
- Televise religious services.
- Provide devotional readings.
- Create parish nurse programs in which nurses within congregations identify and develop a practice that includes home visits to older adults within the church family.

When an individual ages, physical and mental deterioration may necessitate the adaptation of spiritual practices and interventions to meet their unique needs. For example, according to Richards (1990), all aspects of life, including the spiritual, are altered when dementia affects a person, but this does not mean that spiritual needs disappear. The attitude that spiritual needs no longer matter to a person who is confused, suffers from memory loss, or is unable to communicate effectively is inappropriate. Interventions for the confused person can include touch, pictures, faith symbols, and music. These interventions can reach an emotional level that may not be immediately apparent in the traditional sense.

SPIRITUAL ELDERS

Blazer (1991) describes spiritual elders as people who "are perceived to 'understand the nature of things' and to have magic powers" (p. 61). Spiritual elders focus on beginnings and endings, and they create rituals that recognize and celebrate transitions and transformative experiences. For example, they may develop rituals to welcome a child into the world, celebrate the wisdom of the postmenopausal woman, or honor the end of a relationship with a partner or substance.

Healing themselves and others through holistic techniques such as massage, therapeutic touch, and a holistic approach to life that emphasizes positive well-being, spiritual elders often provide natural healing knowledge in a broad, spiritual context that is often a metaphor for self-transformation (Miller, 1995). These are powerful forces that should be recognized and understood, since they can be extremely effective tools for healing.

In Western society, aging individuals who have reached a level of spiritual maturity, or gerotranscendence, will often exhibit different behaviors from their less spiritual contemporaries. Spiritual elders will be more likely to discuss topics other than their health or physical limitations. They often have a different perspective of time, and they might prefer to discuss adventures of the past, the dying process, or how their experiences have shaped their lives. Meditation, solitude, or peaceful reflective times might be more important than at earlier stages of their lives (Wadensten & Carlsson, 2003).

Cultural Wisdom

Culture and spirituality are closely related concepts. Miller (1995) explains that they are often so closely related that it is difficult to distinguish between those aspects of a cultural belief system that arise from a sense of religion/spirituality and those that stem from the ethnic/cultural heritage. Spirituality may be determined entirely by cultural norms, it may be opposed to cultural norms, or it can be influenced by both cultural norms and individual experiences. For example, 75% of Haitians practice voodoo (declared to be the cultural heritage of Haiti by President Aristide in 1991), yet many have converted to Protestant Christianity (in opposition to cultural norms) and have moved to the United States where new experiences temper their beliefs (Martsolf, 1997). All cultures use some form of communication with a Higher Being and may incorporate meditation, prayer, contemplation, or rituals in their spirituality.

For a wide variety of ethnic elders, religion and a sense of spirituality provide support in daily living as well as in times of adversity. However, there are differences among the ethnic and racial groups when it comes to religious involvement. For example, older blacks reported a higher degree of religious involvement than did older whites (Koenig, 1999). The latter may be due to the fact that women's roles in religious practices typically involve social activities, caregiving, and nurturing (Isaia et al., 1999). The aging African American woman's spirituality is often closely tied to personal experiences, interpersonal relationships, and the maintenance of community (Lauver, 2000). Within the African American community, religion is a powerful personal and institutional resource for managing the unique life circumstances, history, and stressors that negatively impact this group (Levin et al., 1994).

Cultural wisdom about health, spirituality, and religion is often the venue of women elders. This information, support, and important health knowledge remain a powerful healing tool for the aging individual. For the Hispanic woman, spirituality is often a blend of Christian beliefs and indigenous influences from the pre- and postcolonial era. The mind, body, and spirit are inseparable and older women are considered wise. They may serve as health practitioners, called parteras or curanderos, and provide information to their community members about health-related issues (Musgrave, Allen, & Allen, 2002).

The Older Woman

Today's older woman is part of a diverse group that varies in income, education level, health, functional abilities, living arrangements, and access to support services. Because women live longer than men, they face unique economic, social, and health challenges.

Gist and Velkoff (1997) note the following statistics:
- Women comprise 55% of all persons aged 60 and over.
- Due to widowhood and the geographic mobility of their children, nearly 80% of older persons who live alone are women.

Aging can be especially difficult for women. Society says that a man becomes more "mature" as he ages but a woman loses her beauty. As a result, body image and anxiety can be major problems for aging women. Spiritual growth for women as they age means they often have to discard society's definition of beauty and youth, which can be a difficult task. However, this "letting go" can be a form of "death" that results in new spiritual life (Fischer, 1998).

Women's spirituality focuses on the value of lived experiences. This spirituality places women at the center, rather than at the margins, of life experience. It strives for the integration of the mind, body, and spirit into a balanced whole (Lauver, 2000). Menopause, for example, may be seen as a psychological, physical, and spiritual event in women's lives. It represents a challenge to a woman's view of herself and the world and, as a result, represents a time when a woman's spiritual beliefs may be challenged. Determining a woman's spiritual beliefs can provide important information about her level of stress during this period in her life (King & Hunter, 2002).

For women, spirituality is associated with positive health outcomes. The spiritual woman experiences improved perception of health, increased rates of positive health behaviors (such as use of mammography), and an increased ability to withstand poverty (Musgrave et al., 2002). Yet, the emerging importance of spirituality and religiosity among women, especially those of various ethnic groups, has received little attention (Levin et al., 1994).

Women experience and express spirituality differently than men (Burkhardt, 1994). Women are consistently found to be more religious than men, and they have a greater likelihood of being church members, praying, attending religious activities, and reading the Bible. Their traditional family-centered roles involve them in behaviors and attitudes that involve nurturing and guidance—behaviors and attitudes that are more consistent with religious practices (Levin et al., 1994). Peace, love, joy, and harmony are not qualities unique to women, but women have often developed these qualities more than men because of their traditional roles and life experiences (Miller, 1995).

Women may value a belief in God or an ultimate being, prayer, meditation, a sense of inner strength, and relationships with others and nature. They often derive more strength from being outdoors and connecting with nature than men do. Women state that spirituality involves the importance of meaning in their lives; influences how they change over time; helps them pay attention to "the quiet inside"; and helps them develop an awareness about the connectedness of events, self, and the process of the life journey (Burkhardt, 1994). This spirituality and religious orientation provide an effective coping method for women during times of stress.

Summary

Spirituality is an integral part of the health and well-being of older adults, especially as they face the many challenges of aging. Religion and spirituality provide men and women with effective strategies for dealing with loss, personal difficulties, stress, illness, surgery, and death. Unique approaches to life can also be learned from the wisdom of spiritual elders.

Key Concepts

1. Spiritual concerns in later life are often driven by the paradoxes of growth/loss and weakness/strength. In the face of these paradoxes, aging individuals can find wisdom, reflection, strength, a sense of purpose, inner peace, and transcendence in their spiritual beliefs.
2. Spirituality in the second half of life involves an ability to think abstractly, tolerate ambiguity and paradox, experience emotional flexibility, and commit to universal values.
3. For many people, sexuality and the expressions of love are also a reflection of spirituality. Most people will maintain their sexual interest and activity well into their advancing age.
4. Many individuals, especially older adults, express their spirituality through their religion and religious practices and behaviors, and most older adults rate religion to be important in their lives.
5. All cultures use some form of communication with a God-force or Higher Being and may incorporate meditation, prayer, contemplation, or rituals in their spirituality.
6. Women experience and express spirituality differently than men, and women are consistently found to be more religious than men.

QUESTIONS FOR REFLECTION

1. The words you use to describe people may indicate your underlying thoughts and feelings about them. Take a few minutes to think about the adjectives you use to describe older and aging individuals. What words come to mind? Are they words that indicate respect, appreciation, or admiration (such as experienced, insightful, and wise)? Or are they words that may indicate a lower or condescending opinion (such as crotchety, shrunken, or cute)?
2. Think about some of the older people you know personally, such as close friends or family members. What are some of the spiritual challenges they face or have faced? What resources could their care providers use to help them deal with these challenges more effectively?

REFERENCES

Adler, L. P. (1995). *Centenarians: The bonus years*. Santa Fe, NM: Health Press.

Ainlay, S. C., & Smith, D. R. (1984). Aging and religious participation. *Journal of Gerontology, 39*(3), 357-363.

Baltes, P. B., & Smith, J. (2003). New frontiers in the future of aging: From successful aging of the young old to the dilemmas of the fourth age. *Gerontology, 49*, 123-135.

Becker, B. (2002). Stage presence—body presence: Movement and body experience with the elderly. *Care Management Journal, 3*(2), 99-106.

Berggren-Thomas, P., & Griggs, M. (1995). Spirituality in aging: Spiritual need or spiritual journey? *Journal of Gerontological Nursing, 21*(3), 5-10.

Blazer, D. (1991). Spirituality and aging well. *Aging Well, 15*(1), 61-65.

Burkhardt, M. A. (1994). Becoming and connecting: Elements of spirituality for women. *Holistic Nursing Practice, 8*(4), 12-21.

Burkhardt, M. A., & Nagai-Jacobson, M. G. (2002). *Spirituality: Living our connectedness*. Albany, NY: Delmar Thomson Learning.

Carson, V. B. (1989). *Spiritual dimensions of nursing practice*. Philadelphia: W. B. Saunders.

Cobb, M., & Robshaw, V. (1998). *The spiritual challenge of health care*. Edinburgh: Churchill Livingstone.

Davenport, B. (2003). Older, wiser, richer—spirituality blooms with age. *Healthwise, 22*(5), 4-5.

Dossey, B. M., Keegan, L., & Guzzetta, C. E. (2000). *Holistic nursing: A handbook for practice* (3rd ed.). Gaithersburg, MD: Aspen.

Ebersole, P., & Hess, P. (1998). *Toward healthy aging: Human needs and nursing response* (5th ed.). St. Louis, MO: Mosby-Year Book.

Ellermann, C. R., & Reed, P. G. (2001). Self-transcendence and depression in middle-age adults. *Western Journal of Nursing Research, 23*(7), 698-713.

Fehring, R. J., Miller, J. F., & Shaw, C. (1997). Spiritual well-being, religiosity, hope, depression, and other mood states in elderly people coping with cancer. *Oncology Nursing Forum, 24*(4), 663-671.

Fischer, K. (1998). *Winter grace: Spirituality and aging*. Nashville: Upper Room Books.

Gist, Y. J., & Velkoff, V. A. (1997). Gender and aging: Demographic dimensions. (U.S. Bureau of the Census International Brief No. 97-3). Retrieved July 26, 2003, from http://www.census.gov/ipc/prod/ib-9703.pdf.

Heintz, L. M. (2001). Spirituality and late adulthood. *Psychological Reports, 88*(3), 651-654.

Hitchcock, J. E., Schubert, P. E., & Thomas, S. A. (1999). *Community health nursing*. New York: Delmar Thomson Learning.

Hunsberger, B. (1985). Religion, age, life satisfaction, and perceived sources of religiousness: A study of older persons. *Journal of Gerontology, 40*(5), 615-620.

Isaia, D., Parker, V., & Murrow, E. (1999). Spiritual well-being among older adults. *Journal of Gerontological Nursing, 25*(8), 16-21.

Kahn, D. J. (1995). Predictors of elderly happiness. *Activities, Adaptation, and Aging, 19*(3), 1-29.

King, D. E., & Hunter, M. H. (2002). Psychologic and spiritual aspects of menopause. *Clinics in Family Practice, 4*(1), 205-220.

Koenig, H. G. (1999). *The healing power of faith.* New York: Simon & Schuster.

Koenig, H. G., George, L. K., & Siegler, I. C. (1988). The use of religion and other emotion-regulating coping strategies among older adults. *Gerontologist, 28*(3), 303-310.

Koenig, H. G., Hays, J. C., Larson, D. B., George, L. K., Cohen, H. J., McCullough, M. E., et al. (1999). Does religious attendance prolong survival? A six-year follow-up study of 3,968 older adults. *Journal of Gerontology: Medical Sciences, 54A*(7), M370-M376.

Krause, N. (1998). Neighborhood deterioration, religious coping, and changes in health during late life. *Gerontologist, 38*(6), 653-664.

Kremer, P. (2002). Spirituality and aging. *Arizona Geriatrics Society Journal, 7*(3), 10-16.

Kübler-Ross, E. (1983). *On children and death.* New York: Touchstone.

Lauver, D. R. (2000). Commonalities in women's spirituality and women's health. *Advanced Nursing Science, 22*(3), 76-88.

Leetun, M. C. (1996). Wellness spirituality in the older adult: Assessment and intervention protocol. *Nurse Practitioner, 21*(8), 60, 65-70.

Lueckenotte, A. G. (2000). *Gerontologic nursing.* St. Louis: Mosby.

Levin, J. S., Taylor, R. J., & Chatters, L. M. (1994). Race and gender differences in religiosity among older adults: Findings from four national surveys. *Journal of Gerontology, 49*(3), S137-S145.

Malcolm, J. (1987). Creative spiritual care for the elderly. *Journal of Christian Nursing, 4*(1), 24-26.

Markides, K. S. (1983). Aging, religiosity, and adjustment: A longitudinal analysis. *Journal of Gerontology, 38*(5), 621-625.

Martsolf, D. S. (1997). Cultural aspects of spirituality in cancer care. *Seminars in Oncology Nursing, 13*(4), 231-236.

McFadden, S. H., & Gerl, R. R. (1990). Approaches to understanding spirituality in the second half of life. *Generations: Aging and the Human Spirit,* 35-38.

Mickley, J., & Soeken, K. (1993). Religiousness and hope in Hispanic- and Anglo-American women with breast cancer. *Oncology Nurses Forum, 20*(8), 1171-1177.

Miller, J. F. (1985). Assessment of loneliness and spiritual well-being in chronically ill and healthy adults. *Journal of Professional Nursing, 1*(2), 79-85.

Miller, M. A. (1995). Culture, spirituality, and women's health. *Journal of Obstetric, Gynecologic, and Neonatal Nursing, 24*(3), 257-263.

Miller, W. R. (Ed.). (1999). *Integrating spirituality into treatment: Resources for practitioners.* Washington, DC: American Psychological Association.

Missinne, L. E. (1990). Death and spiritual concerns of older adults. *Generations: Aging and the Human Spirit,* 45-47.

Mull, C. S., Cox, C. L, & Sullivan, J. A. (1987). Religion's role in the health and well-being of well elders. *Public Health Nursing, 4*(3), 151-159.

Musgrave, C. F., Allen, C. E., & Allen, G. J. (2002). Spirituality and health for women of color. *American Journal of Public Health, 92*(4), 557-560.

O'Brien, M. E. (1999). *Spirituality in nursing: Standing on holy ground.* Boston: Jones & Bartlett.

Post, S. G., Puchalski, C. M., & Larson, D. N. (2000). Physicians and patient spirituality: Professional boundaries, competency, and ethics. *Annals of Internal Medicine, 132*(7), 578-583.

Reed, E. (2002). Sexual intimacy and aging. *Arizona Geriatrics Society Journal, 7*(2), 6-19.

Richards, M. (1990). Meeting the spiritual needs of the cognitively impaired. *Generations: Aging and the Human Spirit*, 63-64.

Schmied, L. A., & Jost, K. J. (1994). Church attendance, religiosity, and health. *Psychological Reports, 74*, 145-146.

Seeber, J. J. (1990). Beginnings of a theology of aging. *Generations: Aging and the Human Spirit*, 48-50.

Strong, J. (1990). An agape experience. *Generations: Aging and the Human Spirit*, 71-72.

Sulmasy, D. P. (1997). *The healer's calling: A spirituality for physicians and other health care professionals.* New York: Paulist Press.

Wadensten, B., & Carlsson, M. (2003). Theory-driven guidelines for practical care of older people, based on the theory of gerotranscendence. *Journal of Advanced Nursing, 41*(5), 462-470.

Young, C. (1993). Spirituality and the chronically ill Christian elderly. *Geriatric Nursing, 14*(6), 298-303.

INDEX

adolescents, spiritual development of, 209–211
advocacy, 36
African Americans
    cultural characteristics of, 81–85
    grief responses of, 194
aging, 221–238
    changing paradigm of, 223
    coping strategies in, 231–232
    health concerns in, 229–230
    hope in, 227
    human spirit and, 223–225
    inner journey of, 224–225
    loss in, 226–227
    love and, 228–229
    religion and, 229–230
    sexuality and, 229
    spiritual assessment in, 114
    spiritual challenges of, 222–223
    spiritual development in, 225–226
    spiritual elders in, 233–235
    spiritual interventions in, 232–233
    transcendence in, 226
    women's situation in, 234–235
AIDS, religion benefits in, 64
air quality, in healing environment, 155–156
Alaskan population. See Native Americans
alienation, spiritual, 117
alternative health care system, 81
American Indians. See Native Americans
anger, spiritual, 118
animal-assisted therapy, 137–142
    animals used in, 141–142
    benefits of, 138–140
    for dying persons, 176
    settings for, 142
    theories on, 138
    types of, 140–141
anticipatory grief, 189–190

anxiety, spiritual, 118
Arab Americans
    cultural characteristics of, 93–94
    death beliefs and practices of, 174
    grief responses of, 194–195
    Islamic religion of, 66–68, 93
aromatherapy, 156, 177
art therapy, 52–53, 130–132, 159, 176
Asian Americans
    cultural characteristics of, 85–88
    death beliefs and practices of, 174
    grief responses in, 193
assessment
    cultural, of self, 78–79
    definition of, 106
    spiritual. See spiritual assessment
attention, to dying person, 175
autonomy, 36
Ayurveda, 87

beliefs and belief systems, 12. See also health
        belief systems
    assessment of, 113–114
    of dying persons, 171
    in grief, 192–195
    related to religion, 65–70
beneficence, 35
biomedical health belief systems, 80
biomedical health care system, 81
biophilic theory
    of animal-assisted therapy, 138
    of environment, 150
blacks/African Americans
    cultural characteristics of, 81–85
    grief responses of, 194
blood pressure, music effects on, 128
body (physical dimension), 5
brainwaves, music effects on, 128

breathing techniques, for meditation, 49
Buddhism, beliefs and practices of, 65–66

cancer
    coping with, in older adults, 232
    religion benefits in, 64
care, spiritual. *See* spiritual care
Catholicism, 68–69
cats, therapy with, 141
chaplains, 27–28
children, 203–219
    psychosocial development of, 205–211
    spiritual assessment of, 210, 212
    spiritual care of, 213–214
        with chronic illness, 214–216
        in dying, 216–217
    spiritual development of, 204–211
    spiritual distress in, 212–213
Chinese Americans. *See* Asian Americans
Chinese medicine, 87
Christianity, beliefs and practices of, 68–69
chromotherapy, 151–152
chronic illness
    in children, 214–216
    in older adults, 231–232
    religion benefits in, 64
clergy, 28–29
color, in healing environment, 151–152
comfort (palliative) care, 180–182, 216–217
communication
    in animal-assisted therapy, 139
    in dying, 173
    in palliative care, 180–181
    transcultural (culturally competent),
        94–95, 195
compassion, 78, 173, 175
complementary (alternative) health care system, 81
confidentiality, 36
connectedness, as spirituality element, 11
coping
    in aging, 231
    with grief, 195
coping humor, 136
counseling, grief, 195–197
Creator, concept of, 4
cultural groups, 81–94
    Arab Americans, 93–94, 174, 194–195
    Asian Americans, 85–88, 174, 193
    blacks/African Americans, 82–85, 194
    Hispanic Americans, 88–90, 173, 193–194
    Native Americans, 90–92, 173–174, 194
    variation among, 82

wisdom in, 233–234
culturally competent care
    for children, 205
    compassion in, 78
    in dying, 173
    in grief, 192–195
    language and, 94–95
    self-assessment for, 78–79
culture
    aging views and, 223
    definition of, 76–78
    end-of-life considerations and, 172–174
    health belief systems of, 79–81
    health care systems related to, 81
curanderos, 31–32, 89
curing, vs. healing, 15
cymatics, 127

dance therapy, 132–134
death. *See* dying and death
design considerations, for healing environment, 150–151, 159–161
despair, spiritual, 118
determinism, 80
development, spiritual, 13–14
    in aging individuals, 225–226
    in children, 204–211
diagnoses, spiritual, 116–118
disability, animal assistance for, 139–140
disenfranchised grief, 190
disequilibrium, spiritual, 9
distress, spiritual, 9, 116–117, 212–213
documentation, of spiritual care, 120
dogs, therapy with, 141
Dossey Spiritual Assessment Tool, 114–115
dying and death, 169–184
    cultural considerations in, 172–174
    grief in. *See* grief
    at home, 181
    hospice care in, 179, 181, 182
    palliative care in, 180–182, 216–217
    psychological dimensions in, 171–172
    religion benefits in, 64
    social dimensions in, 172
    spiritual care in, 174–178
        for children, 216–217
        healing strategies in, 176–177
        interactions with persons in, 175
        at moment of death, 178
        reflection in, 177
        rituals in, 177–178
    spiritual dimensions in, 170–171

elderly persons. *See* Aging
elders, spiritual, 233–235
electromagnetic radiation, in healing environment, 153–155
end-of-life care. *See* dying and death; grief
endorphins, music effects on, 128
environment
    for dying persons, 175, 177–178
    for spiritual assessment, 110–111
    for spiritual healing, 147–164
        air quality in, 155
        color in, 151–152
        description of, 148–149
        design considerations in, 150–151
        furnishings in, 158–159
        health care provider as, 161
        historical view of, 149–150
        lighting in, 153–155
        natural elements in, 152–153
        noise control in, 156–158
        smells in, 156
        temperature in, 155–156
        wayfinding in, 159–161
Erikson's psychosocial stages, 206–211
ethical issues, in spiritual care, 33–37
evaluating, spiritual care, 119–120
expressions, of spirituality, 12–13. *See also specific types*

faith
    assessment of, 113–114
    definition of, 12
    development of, 13–14, 204–211
    of health care providers, 32–33
    types of, 13–14
family
    death of child in, 217
    of dying person, spiritual dimensions of, 171
    importance of
        to Asian Americans, 86–88
        to Hispanic Americans, 89–90
    photos of, for dying persons, 176
    as spiritual care provider, 30
FICA Model of Spiritual Assessment, 113–114
flowers, in healing environment, 152–153, 158–159
folk healers, 30–32, 81
    in black/African American culture, 84–85
    in Hispanic American culture, 89
    in Native American culture, 91–92
formal spiritual assessment, 112–116
Fowler's stages of faith development, 13–14, 206–211, 225

friends, as spiritual care providers, 30
furnishings, in healing environment, 158–159

gallows humor, 136
gardens
    healing effects of, 152–153
    memory, 176
God
    concept of, 4
    as spirituality element, 9 10
gratitude, 50–51
Greek Orthodox beliefs and practices, 69
grief, 187–199
    acute, 189
    anticipatory, 189–190
    characteristics of, 189
    chronic, 189
    communication in, 195
    coping with, 195
    counseling on, 195–197
    culturally different responses in, 192–195
    definition of, 188–189
    disenfranchised, 190
    healing in, 195–197
    normal responses in, 190–192
    in palliative care, 181
    physical symptoms of, 191
    psychological responses to, 190–191
    social changes in, 191–192
    spiritual dimensions of, 192
growth, spiritual, 14. *See also* development, spiritual
guided imagery, 50
guilt, spiritual, 118

healing
    cultural views of, 77
    definition of, 15–16, 77
    for dying persons, 176–177
    environment for. *See* environment, for spiritual healing
    folk. *See* folk healers
    in grief, 195–197
    prayer in, 47. *See also* prayer
    rituals in, 55. *See also* rituals
    spiritual presence in, 17–18
    therapeutic interventions for. *See* therapeutic interventions
health
    problems with, in older adults, 229–230
    spiritual, 16–17

health belief systems, 79–81
    of Arab Americans, 93–94
    of Asian Americans, 86–88
    of blacks/African Americans, 84–85
    of Hispanic Americans, 89–90
    of Native Americans, 91–92
health care definitions, of spirituality, 8–9
health care providers
    cultural self-assessment of, 78–79
    faith of, 32–33
    as healing environments, 161
    prayer by, 47–48
    spiritual care by, 25–26
    spiritual self-assessment of, 78–79
health care systems, 81
hearing, at death, 178
heartbeat, music effects on, 128
Higher Power, concept of, 4
Hinduism, beliefs and practices of, 66
hippotherapy, 142
Hispanic Americans
    cultural characteristics of, 88–90
    death beliefs and practices of, 173
    grief responses in, 193–194
HIV/AIDS, religion benefits in, 64
holistic health belief systems, 80–81
home environment
    dying in, 181
    in health care setting, 158–159
hope
    aging and, 227
    as spirituality element, 11
horses, therapy with, 142
hospice care, 179, 181, 182
Howden's Spirituality Assessment Scale, 113
humor therapy, 134–137

immune function, music effects on, 129
implementing, spiritual care, 119
incongruity theory, of humor, 135
infants
    spiritual care of, 213
    spiritual development of, 205–206, 211
informal spiritual assessment, 112
inspiriting, 9
Islam
    beliefs and practices of, 66–68, 93
    death beliefs and practices in, 174
    grief responses in, 194–195

Japanese Americans. See Asian Americans
JAREL Spiritual Well-Being Scale, 114

Joint Commission on Accreditation of Health-
    care Organizations, spiritual assess-
    ment guidelines of, 107
journal writing, by dying person, 176
joy, spiritual, 62
Judaism
    beliefs and practices of, 68, 69
    death beliefs and practices in, 174

language, culturally competent care and,
    94–95
Latinos
    cultural characteristics of, 88–90
    death beliefs and practices of, 173
    grief responses of, 93–194
laughter therapy, 134–137
lighting, in healing environment, 153–155, 178
loss
    in aging, 226
    grief in. See grief
    spiritual, 118
love, aging and, 238–239

magicoreligious health belief systems, 80
materialism, objective, 80
meaning, as spirituality element, 10
mechanistic view, of health beliefs, 80
medical theories, of spirituality, 5–6
medicine men and women, 31–32
meditation, 48–50
mentors, spiritual, 30
Mexican Americans. See Hispanic Americans
mind (psychological dimension), 5
    in dying, 171–172
moral issues, in spiritual care, 34–35
movement therapy, 132–134
muscle tension, music effects on, 128
music therapy, 126–130, 158
    benefits of, 129
    for dying persons, 176
    interventions in, 130
    physiological responses in, 127–129
    principles of, 127
Muslim beliefs and practices, 66–68, 93
    on death, 174
    in grief, 194–195

Native Americans
    cultural characteristics of, 90–92
    death beliefs and practices of, 173–174
    grief responses of, 194
    healing environments of, 149

nature
    in healing environment, 152–153
    spending time in, 51–52
needs, spiritual, 9
Neuman (Betty) systems model, 6
Newman's (Margaret) theory of health, 6
noise control, in healing environment, 156–158
nonmaleficence, 36
nurses, as spiritual care providers, 25–26, 29–30
nursing theories, of spirituality, 6–7

objective materialism, 80
older adults. *See* Aging
others, as spirituality element, 9–10

pain, spiritual, 9, 117
palliative care, 180–182, 216–217
parish nurses, 29–30
Parse (Rosemary) theory of human becoming, 6
pet therapy. *See* animal-assisted therapy
physical dimension (body), 5
physical symptoms, of grief, 191
physicians, as spiritual care providers, 26
physiological responses
    to laughter, 135–136
    to music therapy, 127–129
Piaget's cognitive phases, 206–211
planning, spiritual care, 118–119
plants, in environment, healing effects of, 152–153
pollution
    air, in healing environment, 155–156
    noise, 156–158
popular health care systems, 81
practice, spiritual. *See* spiritual practice
prayer, 45–48
    definition of, 45–46
    in grief, 197
    healing effects of, 47
    by health care providers, 47–48
    techniques for, 46
    types of, 46–47
Protestantism, 68–69
psychological dimension (mind), 5
    in dying, 171–172
psychological response, to grief, 190–191
psychological theory, of spirituality, 5
pulse rate, music effects on, 128
purpose, as spirituality element, 10

qualitative spiritual assessment tools, 115–116
quality of life, spiritual, 9

reason, in spiritual care, 105
reductionism, 80
reflection
    in dying, 177
    in spiritual care, 105
relatedness, as spirituality element, 11
relationships
    changes of, in grief, 191–192
    with dying person, 175
    provider-client, for spiritual assessment, 109–110
    in spiritual care, 105
release theory, of humor, 135
religion, 59–72
    aging and, 229–232
    beliefs and practices of, 12
        Buddhism, 65–66
        Christianity, 68–69
        Hinduism, 66
        integrating into health care, 69–70
        Islam, 66–68, 174
        Judaism, 68, 69, 174
    of cultural groups
        Arab Americans, 93
        Asian Americans, 86
        blacks/African Americans, 83
        Hispanic Americans, 88
        Native Americans, 91
    definition of, 60–61, 105
    development of, in children, 204–211
    health effects of, 15–16, 61–64
    music in, 126
    vs. spirituality, 59–60
religiosity, definition of, 60–61
respiration, music effects on, 128
restoration, in spiritual care, 105
rheumatoid arthritis, religion benefits in, 64
rituals, 43–57
    art, 52–53, 159, 176
    creating, 44–45
    description of, 43–44
    for dying persons, 177–178
    gratitude, 50–51
    guided imagery, 50
    healing force of, 55
    meditation, 48–50
    in nature, 51–52
    prayer, 44–48, 197
    sacred, 44

secular, 44
self-generated, 44
storytelling, 53–55
traditional, 44
visualization, 49

sacred spaces, for spiritual assessment, 110–111
sadness, in grief, 190–191
scientific health belief systems, 80
self, as spirituality element, 9–10
self-assessment
    cultural, 78–79
    spiritual, 108–109
self-care, spiritual, 109
senses, of dying persons, 177–178
sexuality, aging and, 239
shamans, 31
shock, in grief, 191
sight, of meaningful objects, for dying persons, 178
signs, in buildings, 161
smells
    for dying persons, 177
    in healing environment, 156
social animals, 140
social changes, in grief, 191–192
social dimensions, of dying, 172
social support, animals and, 139
social workers, as spiritual care providers, 26
sociological theory, of spirituality, 5
sound
    control of, in healing environment, 156–158
    in meditation, 49
    principles of, for music therapy, 127
Spanish Americans. See Hispanic Americans
spiritual assessment
    of children, 210, 212
    conducting, 111–112
    definition of, 106
    formal, 112–115
    framework for, 115–116
    importance of, 106–107
    informal, 112
    interdisciplinary team for, 108
    models for, 112–116
    organizational mandates for, 107–108
    preparing for, 108–111
    provider-client relationship establishment for, 109–110
    qualitative tools for, 115–116
    sacred space for, 110–111
    of self, 78–79, 108–109

timing of, 110
Spiritual Assessment Tool (Dossey), 114–115
spiritual care, 23–40
    barriers to, 33–34
    for children, 213–217
    definition of, 104–105
    documentation of, 120
    at end of life. See dying and death; grief
    ethical issues in, 34–37
    evaluating, 119–120
    implementing, 119
    interdisciplinary team for, 108
    moral issues in, 34–35
    for older adults, 232–233
    planning, 118–119
    of self, 109
    systematic approach to, 105
spiritual care providers
    spirituality of, 32–33
    types of, 24–32
        generalists, 25–26
        specialists, 27–32
spiritual diagnoses, 116–118
spiritual dimension, 4–5
    in dying and death, 170–171
    in grief, 182
spiritual disequilibrium, 9
spiritual distress, 9, 116–117, 212–213
spiritual elders, 233–235
spiritual health, 16–17
spiritual issues, 8
spiritual needs, 9
spiritual pain, 9, 117
spiritual practice
    of Arab Americans, 93
    of Asian Americans, 86
    of blacks/African Americans, 83
    of Hispanic Americans, 88
    of Native Americans, 91
    vs. rituals, 43–44
spiritual well-being, 9, 16–17
spirituality
    definition of, 7–9, 77
    elements of, 9–13
    vs. religion, 59–60
storytelling, 53–55
stress
    laughter and, 136
    music effects on, 129
    from poorly designed buildings, 160
superiority theory, of humor, 135
surgery, coping with, in older adults, 231

taste, for dying persons, 177–178
team approach
    to palliative care, 180–181
    to spiritual care, 108
temperature
    body, music effects on, 128
    in healing environment, 155–156
terminal illness. *See* dying and death; grief
theological theory, of spirituality, 5
theories
    on animal-assisted therapy, 138
    on humor, 135
    of spirituality, 5–7
therapeutic interventions, 125–145
    animal-assisted, 137–142
    art, 52–53, 130–132, 159, 176
    dance, 132–134
    humor, 134–137

    movement, 132–134
    music, 126–130, 158, 176
touch, for dying persons, 177
traditional medical systems, 81, 87
transcendence, in aging, 226

ultraviolet light, in healing environment,
    153–155

values, 35
visualization, in meditation, 49

Watson (Jean) theory of human caring, 7
wayfinding, 159–161
well-being, spiritual, 9, 16–17
wisdom, cultural, 233–234
women, older, 234–235